Food 4 Osteoporosis
Four Week Eating Plan
Volume 2
First Edition

Fight Osteoporosis with Food

By Nancy Robinson, Registered Dietitian Nutritionist

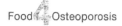

Also available by Nancy Robinson RDN

Food 4 Osteoporosis Four Week Eating Plan Volume 1

Contents

Introduction

The Primary Goal of the Food 4 Osteoporosis Four Week Eating Plan is to provide your bones with nutrients from meals that contain lots of fruits and vegetables and only moderate amounts of meat and cheese.   A high vegetable and fruit intake provides micronutrients that are essential for bone formation.   Fruits and vegetables contain more of the key nutrients necessary for bone strength than animal foods.   Vegetable intake is key to obtaining calcium from a variety of plant sources.   Vegetables and fruits also reduce the acid load of the diet.

A large number of studies show that as fruit and vegetable consumption increases so does bone density.   It is possible that fruits and vegetables are beneficial to bone health through yet to be discovered mechanisms.   Amy Joy Lanou, Ph.D. and Michael Castleman in their book "Building Bone Vitality" reviewed 103 studies on the bone mineral density effects of fruits and vegetables or studies of nutrients found mainly in fruits and vegetables. Eighty four percent of the studies found that with an increase in fruit, vegetable or anti-oxidant intake bone mineral density also increased.   Nine percent of the studies were inconclusive and only 7 percent showed no effect on bone mineral density from fruits and vegetables.

In addition to being crucial for healthy bones, a liberal fruit and vegetable intake may also reduce your risk of developing other diseases such as cancer, diabetes, heart disease and Alzheimer's.

Beverages
You can drink coffee or tea on the Eating Plan but it is recommended that you limit servings to one to two cups (caffeinated or decaffeinated) per day if not contraindicated for other health reasons.   Some studies have shown that excess intake of coffee seems to increase renal calcium loss.   However, another study concluded 1 to 2 cups of coffee per day has little impact on calcium loss.

It is also recommended that you avoid soft drinks, diet or regular, and other sweetened beverages. Studies on the effect of drinking sodas and bone health have conflicting findings with some results indicating problems, others finding no negative effects and others yielding uncertain results.   One Tufts University study only saw a problem with cola drinks in women and not with non-cola drinks like Sprite® and Mountain Dew®.   Cola drinks generally contain the additive phosphoric acid and Sprite® and Mountain Dew® do not. Some recent research has found an association between sugar-sweetened sodas and accelerated cellular aging of tissues.

Herbal teas, rooibos tea and hibiscus tea are good beverage choices.   Water with lemon/lime juice or mineral water is great for adding alkalinity to the diet. Be sure to drink lots of fluids throughout the day.

Alcohol
Some researchers believe moderate alcohol intake is not harmful to bone but that chronic alcohol abuse is detrimental to bone health, with one of the mechanisms being a direct toxic effect on bone forming cells. Whether to consume alcohol is a personal decision. If you choose to drink alcohol, then like so many other things in life, moderation is best.

Substitutions
In order to take advantage of local and seasonal availability and variety as well as personal food preferences you may substitute different fruits and vegetables for the fruits and vegetables specified in the Eating plan. You can always eat more vegetables. Focus on eating a variety of fruits and vegetables.

The Eating Plan is designed to start on Monday (Day 1) however you may switch the days around and repeat days if you don't like the Eating plan for that particular day. You may switch the lunch and dinner for the day. If you don't want to cook every day then on some days make enough for more than one day and eat leftovers. The menus are designed to have the more time consuming recipes on the weekend.

If you can't tolerate any milk products you may substitute non-diary yogurt for Greek yogurt. Choose one containing 300 mg. calcium per 1 cup serving. Greek yogurt is high in protein (23 g. protein/cup) and substituting a non-dairy yogurt will probably give you less protein. See the "Protein needs for strength training" chart in the

Appendix (p. 157) for ideas on how to replace the protein lost when choosing a non-dairy yogurt. You may substitute another plant milk for the almond milk. If possible, choose one containing 300 mg. calcium per 1 cup serving.

You may use rolled oats instead of steel cut oats if you prefer rolled.

Acid Load
Each day's menu includes enough bone healthy fruits and vegetables to balance out the high acid foods in that day's menu. A popular theory related to osteoporosis and diet is that the higher the acid load or acid producing potential of your diet the harder the body has to work to maintain a healthy blood pH. This is considered an even more significant issue in older people because of declining kidney function. The theory proposes that the body tries to defend against increasing acid by breaking down bone and muscle. Some scientists believe dietary acid loads from Western diets may be a risk factor for osteoporosis. The acid load of a particular food is determined by what the food releases into the bloodstream upon metabolism not on the acidity of the food prior to metabolism. Grains like breads, cereals, rice, and pasta as well as meat, fish, egg yolks and cheeses release acids into the bloodstream upon metabolism. Fruits and vegetables break down to add alkali (opposite of acid) to the bloodstream which helps neutralize acid. Sugars and fats are generally neutral. Foods with higher acid loads, such as cheese and meat, don't have to be eliminated from the diet but they need to be eaten in moderation and correctly balanced with alkaline foods so the net effect is a more alkaline, bone healthy diet.

Research indicates the best way to reduce dietary acid load is to eat lots of fruits and vegetables with modest amounts of breads, cereals and pastas and adequate protein but not excessive animal protein.

Follow my Blog at www.food4osteoporosis.com for updates on studies and new information related to the osteoporosis acid load theory.

Calcium
Each day's menu has approximately 1200 milligrams of calcium. If you follow the menu plan it is not necessary or beneficial to take a calcium supplement. If you want to avoid dairy products then use a

non-dairy yogurt when yogurt is included on the menu. Use a yogurt product with 300 milligrams calcium per 8 ounce serving. Calcium absorption is highest in amounts less than 500 milligrams of calcium at one time which is why the Eating Plan often has you divide the smoothies in half so that you drink them at two different times of the day.

It is definitely important that we all get adequate calcium however recent studies have questioned the safety of taking large doses of calcium supplements. The results of studies dealing with the risks and positive effects of calcium have been very inconsistent however they do seem to indicate that getting all your calcium as one or two large doses of a supplement is not the way the body is designed to absorb calcium and is not the same as getting your calcium from food. So with calcium more may not be better. Calcium from supplements may increase the risk of cardiovascular disease and kidney stones if you get too much calcium from supplements or if you already get enough calcium from your diet and take supplemental calcium. Calcium supplements are thought to cause blood calcium levels to increase much more abruptly than calcium rich foods. Mark Hegsted, a long time Harvard nutrition researcher, who died in 2009 at age 95, suggested that very high calcium intakes consumed for many years impaired the body's ability to regulate calcium resulting in a disruption of calcium absorption and excretion.

Regarding the increased risk of cardiovascular disease due to calcium supplements, the theory has been proposed that giving large amounts of calcium as supplements at one time may be facilitating the development of calcifications in the arteries. In the Women's Health Initiative study the women consuming more calcium from their diets were less likely to develop kidney stones so dietary calcium may act differently in regard to kidney stone formation than calcium supplements. Since calcium from food is absorbed at a slower rate than from supplements and usually in smaller amounts, at this point it seems safest to get your calcium from food instead of supplements.

Some research suggests that it may be healthier to get calcium from a variety of plant foods because they contain other important bone building nutrients. While calcium is necessary to good bone health, the strength of your bones depends more on everything you eat and how active you are than just how much calcium you consume.

Countries with the highest consumption of milk, dairy and calcium have the world's highest fracture rates. Many non-western countries with the lowest fracture rates and osteoporosis consume less calcium than western countries (400 to 600 milligrams per day). Explanations for this "Calcium Paradox" may relate to what else these populations are consuming in their diets and the significant differences between western and non-western diets in intakes of processed foods, sodium, meat, dairy, fruits and vegetables.

Smoothies
Some days the smoothie is split between 2 meals or a meal and a snack. This is necessary to distribute protein and calcium for maximum absorption and utilization.

You may add water or ice cubes if a different consistency is desired. It is fine to substitute different fruits in the smoothie recipes and you may use fresh, frozen or canned fruit. If you have an oversupply of ripe bananas - peel, slice, wrap in plastic wrap and freeze for use later. If you have parsley or other greens that you need to use before they go bad then add them to your smoothie rather than let them go to waste. The flax seed is optional and something you should transition to if you are not used to a high fiber diet.

When the smoothie recipe calls for Greek yogurt the calcium calculation is based on a yogurt containing 300 mg. calcium per 1 cup serving (Nutrition label will say 30% of the Daily value for calcium). When the recipe calls for almond milk the calcium calculation is based on almond milk containing 300 mg. calcium per 1 cup serving (or 30% of the calcium Daily value). If using a plant milk product containing more than 300 mg. calcium then use only the amount of milk required for 300 mg calcium and use water for the rest of the liquid, if needed.

Salt/Sodium
The sodium content of the menus is approximately 1500 milligrams or less per day to accommodate individuals who need or want to limit sodium intake. If the menu is below 1500 milligrams for that particular day the plan will tell you how much additional salt you can

add to food or in preparing the recipes (beyond what is already in the recipe) that day and still be within 1500 milligrams sodium. Each daily menu also states how much additional salt you can add to food and not exceed 2300 milligrams per day.

Your use of salt should be determined according to your specific situation.   High sodium/salt intakes may be a risk factor for numerous health conditions. The Dietary Guidelines for Americans recommends limiting sodium to less than 2300 milligrams per day or 1500 milligrams if you are 51 years or older, if you are Black or you have high blood pressure, diabetes or chronic kidney disease. The American Heart Association recommends 1500 mg. sodium per day. Each 1/8 teaspoon of salt added in cooking or directly to food adds 291 milligrams of sodium.   A few studies have investigated the effect of sodium on bone density. The results have been mixed with some indicating a high salt diet reduces bone density and some finding no effect on bone density. One of the main sources of sodium in the American diet is processed food. Restaurant food can also be a significant source of sodium.

Calories
All daily menus contain approximately 1600 calories to accommodate individuals trying to lose or maintain their weight. If you are not trying to lose weight or restrict your calories to 1600 per day you may:
- Use more of the heart healthy fats such as olive oil, almond butter, avocado and nuts, however you should still limit these fats to moderate amounts.
- Be more generous with the salad dressings.
- Eat more fruits and vegetables or add more fruits or vegetables to the Smoothies.
- Add a few squares of a high cocoa content chocolate bar for dessert. Try to go with an 85% or higher cocoa content and preferably not one containing additives such as soy.

Each day's menu outlines additional food options specific to that day for those not limiting calories to 1600 per day. The sodium level will go up with the extra food so if you are limiting sodium you may need to decrease salt with the larger portion sizes.

When restricted to 1600 calories the Eating Plan does not contain enough calories for pregnant or lactating women or for growing children.

With daily exercise and moderate sensible eating most people should be able to stay at a healthy weight. When you occasionally overeat or overindulge in high calorie foods either adjust your eating afterward to compensate or plan ahead by cutting back on some other food. Read food labels and learn where excess calories slip in and how to compensate without sacrificing good nutrition. Calorie counting does work as a weight loss strategy but as one transitions from weight loss mode to weight maintenance mode it is much more enjoyable to exercise daily and practice moderation and restraint in eating rather than worrying with counting calories.

Protein
The menus average 75 to 80 grams of protein per day, evenly distributed throughout the day, which is the best way to get your protein. If you currently eat only cereal for breakfast you probably aren't getting enough protein at breakfast. The eating plan will ensure you get your morning protein. In general there is an upper limit on how much protein can be used for muscle synthesis at one time so there is no advantage to consuming more than 25 to 30 grams of protein at one time. Your protein requirement will be higher if you are engaged in a strength-training program to build muscle and strengthen your bones. See Appendix A, page 156, for guidelines on meeting your protein needs when strength training.

If you have a specific condition affecting protein metabolism work with a dietitian specializing in that condition.

Fat
The fat content of the menus, when limited to 1600 calories per day, is low to moderate depending on the day and predominately from food containing heart healthy fats such as olive oil, fish, nuts, almond butter and avocado. If calories are not restricted to 1600 per day, and heart healthy fats are chosen, then the fat content of the menus may be higher, depending on the foods eaten, but still healthy. Cheese and meat servings are small in size to limit unhealthy fats and acid load yet still allow enjoyment of these foods.

Fiber
The menus are high in fiber, which is good for digestive and heart health and may facilitate weight loss by filling you up and keeping you from feeling hungry. You need to drink plenty of fluids when consuming a high fiber diet. If you currently do not eat a high fiber diet you should transition yourself gradually on to the high fiber intake to avoid bloating, gas or discomfort as your body adjusts to the higher fiber intake.

Choosing whole grain bread or crackers
Read the label. Manufacturers must list their ingredients in descending order, so the first few ingredients are key. When purchasing whole grain breads, crackers or chips the word "whole" should be on the ingredient list. The first ingredient should be "whole wheat flour" or whatever whole grains the product contains. The terms "stone ground", "cracked wheat", "multigrain", "whole grain", "wheat or wheat flour" do not prove the product is 100% whole grain. If a product has the 100% Whole Grains Stamp on it then all its grain ingredients are whole grains. Even if it is 100% whole grains, it can still contain high fructose corn syrup or be high in sugar or hydrogenated fat so look for these ingredients as well. Also be sure the label does not include a long list of additives. Usually, a good guideline is the fewer ingredients, the better.

There are two Whole Grain Stamps, the basic stamp and the 100% whole grain stamp. If a product has the 100% Whole Grains Stamp on it then all its grain ingredients are whole grains and it has at least 16 g of whole grains per serving. The Basic stamp has at least 8 g of whole grains per serving but may contain refined grains. The recommended number of grams per serving is 16 g, and the recommended number of whole grain grams per day is 48 g.

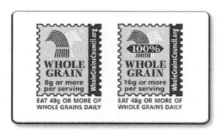

Courtesy Oldways and the Whole Grains Council
wholegrainscouncil.org

Tips
Many stores (Whole Foods, Trader Jo's, local health food stores and larger regional grocery stores) now carry the specialty flours (garbanzo bean, teff, almond meal/flour) required for the muffins or you can order them from specialty flour companies such as Bob's Red Mill at www.bobsredmill.com

For recipes, the serving size is indicated in the recipe by the number of servings. Snacks can be eaten anytime of the day.

Other considerations
If you are accustomed to eating high fat, high sodium processed foods or very few fruits and vegetables then you may find that you need to give yourself some time to adjust to a different and healthier way of eating. If you stick with it you will come to appreciate the greater variety of flavors and positive experiences of eating nutritious, real food that is good for your bones, body and mind.

If you take the anticoagulant warfarin and the Food 4 Osteoporosis Eating Plan is higher in vegetables, especially kale and other green leafy vegetables, than you are used to eating, then work with your health care provider to monitor and adjust your medication as appropriate.

If you are a menstruating woman then the diet may not meet your iron requirements and you should discuss the use of an iron supplement with your health care provider. An iron supplement should not be necessary, and in general is not recommended due to possible adverse effects of excess iron, for women no longer menstruating or for men unless you have a unique health situation warranting iron supplementation.

The Eating Plan is not a substitute for individualized care by a physician. Individuals with additional health challenges and complications including, but not limited to diabetes, kidney disease, cancer, irritable bowel syndrome or celiac disease should work directly with a Registered Dietitian Nutritionist that specializes in these conditions.

Don't Forget the Primary Goal of the Eating Plan is to provide your bones with nutrients from meals that contain lots of fruits and vegetables and only moderate amounts of meat and cheese.

To download the weekly grocery list as a PDF or Excel file that you can further customize to your own shopping needs go to www.food4osteoporosis.com/grocery-lists.html or download on your Smartphone.

An Online Eating Plan with menus and recipes for every day of the year is available by subscription.   To access the plan go to www.food4osteoporosis.com and click on the "online program" tab at the top right hand side of the page. The Online Plan always offers the most up to date osteoporosis nutrition information and 4 weeks of menus, recipes and color photos, which change weekly.   New recipes, guidelines and osteoporosis nutrition information are added regularly.   The Online Food 4 Osteoporosis Eating Plan also includes sections on "What to do with Leftovers" and a "Time Saving Menu Guide".   A free demo with access to one weeks worth of menus is available.   There is a 3 month and 12 month subscription option.

For more information on fighting osteoporosis with food, when future volumes of the Four Week Eating Plans will be available and to follow my blog go to www.food4osteoporosis.com

You can follow Food 4 Osteoporosis on Pinterest at www.pinterest.com/food4osteopor/

If you have suggestions for improving future Eating Plan volumes or other input regarding how the Food 4 Osteoporosis Four Week Eating Plans can help you fight osteoporosis I welcome and appreciate your ideas, which can be communicated to me at nancy@food4osteoporosis.com

Day 1 Menu

Breakfast
Ricotta English Muffin with Sliced Strawberries
1 Egg cooked any way
Beverage of Choice

Lunch
Hummus
Raw Vegetables
Whole Grain Crackers or Bread
Pineapple with Spicy Yogurt
Beverage of Choice

Dinner
Eggplant with Barley and Yogurt Topping
Mixed Green Salad with Parsley Dill Dressing
Chocolate Covered Strawberries
Beverage of Choice

If restricting sodium to 1500 mg/day: Do not add additional salt to food or in cooking beyond what is already in the recipes - reduce salt in the Eggplant recipe from ¼ tsp. to 1/8 tsp.
2300 mg/day: May add an additional generous 1/4 tsp. salt to food or in cooking.

If not restricting calories to 1600/day:
Lunch: May have more Hummus and Vegetables and Pineapple Yogurt.
Dinner: May have more Eggplant, a serving of whole grain bread and additional chocolate covered strawberries.

Recipes:
Breakfast: English Muffin with Ricotta Cheese and Sliced Strawberries, 1 Egg cooked as desired.

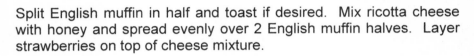

For each person:
1 Whole grain English muffin
½ cup ricotta cheese
1 tsp. honey
4 medium strawberries, sliced

Split English muffin in half and toast if desired. Mix ricotta cheese with honey and spread evenly over 2 English muffin halves. Layer strawberries on top of cheese mixture.

Nutritional analysis per serving: 342 calories, 20 g. protein, 5 g. fiber, 11 g. fat, 520 mg. calcium, 396 mg. sodium.

Lunch: Hummus with Raw Vegetables and Crackers, Pineapple with Spicy Yogurt.

You can make your own homemade hummus or purchase it already made. Try a variety of brands to determine which one you like best.

Per person:
1/2 cup Hummus with as many raw vegetables as you like.
Try: Broccoli, cauliflower, carrot sticks, cucumbers, red pepper slices or any other vegetable that sounds good to you.
Plus 6 whole grain crackers (I like Flackers – crackers made from flax seeds or try Multigrain Wasa Flatbreads) or a slice of whole grain bread.

Pineapple with Spicy Yogurt recipe:

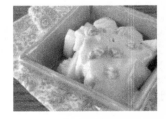

Per person:
¼ cup non-fat, plain Greek Yogurt
1 tsp. 100% maple syrup
1/8 tsp. cinnamon
1/8 tsp. ginger
1/8 tsp. allspice
½ cup pineapple chunks
Chopped walnuts for top, if not limiting calories to 1600/day

Mix yogurt, maple syrup, cinnamon, ginger and allspice until well blended.   Spoon over pineapple chunks.   Top with chopped walnuts, if not limiting calories to 1600/day.

Possible spice substitutions or additions include cardamom or anise.

Nutritional analysis per serving without walnuts: 87 calories, 6 g. protein, 1 g. fiber, 0 fat, 90 mg. calcium, 25 mg. sodium.

Dinner: Eggplant with Bulgur and Yogurt Topping, Mixed Green Salad with Parsley Dressing, Chocolate Covered Strawberries

Eggplant Recipe: Makes 2 servings.   1 serving is ½ of an eggplant.
Preheat oven to 350° F.

1 Eggplant
2 tsp. olive oil
1 tsp. garlic powder
2 tsp. ground cumin
2 tsp. ground coriander
1/8 tsp. cayenne pepper – use more if you like a lot of heat
1 tsp. smoked paprika
½ cup raw bulgur wheat
1 cup water
2 Tbsp. raisins
2 Tbsp. slivered almonds
2 green onions, chopped
1 Tbsp. lemon juice
¼ tsp. sea salt – if limiting sodium to 1500 mg./day reduce salt to
    1/8 tsp.
¼ cup Italian parsley, chopped

1 cup plain, non-fat Greek Yogurt
¼ tsp. sea salt
2 Tbsp. slivered almonds

Cut stem end off eggplant. Cut eggplant in half lengthwise. Being careful not to slice through to the skin, score the flesh of each eggplant half with crisscrossed lines so that it will scoop out more readily into bite-sized pieces once cooked. Brush flesh of eggplant halves with olive oil.

In small bowl mix garlic, cumin, coriander, cayenne pepper and smoked paprika. Spread spice mixture evenly over eggplant halves, rubbing it into the surface and cracks where you made the crisscross lines. Place on a baking sheet and bake at 350° for 50 to 60 minutes or until eggplant is soft.

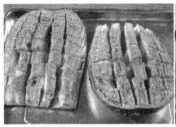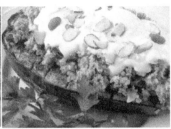

Mix ½ cup bulgur with 1 cup water in a saucepan and bring to a boil. Then reduce heat to low and cook covered 15 minutes or until done. Once bulgur is done add raisins, almonds, green onions, lemon juice, ¼ tsp. sea salt and parsley to bulgur and mix well. Keep covered and warm until ready to add to eggplant.

Mix Greek Yogurt with ¼ tsp. sea salt. When eggplant is done add ½ of bulgur mixture to top of each eggplant half and top with ½ cup yogurt mixture per eggplant half. Sprinkle 1 Tbsp. slivered almonds, per eggplant half, on top of yogurt.

Nutritional Analysis per serving: 534 calories, 27 g. protein, 23 g. fiber, 21 g. fat, 365 mg calcium, 657 mg. sodium. (If reduce salt to 1/8 tsp. then sodium is 512 mg./serving).

Mixed Greens Salad with Parsley Dill Dressing Recipe:

To make salad mix ½ cup cherry or sliced tomatoes and at least 1 cup mixed greens (may use more than 1 cup) per person. Buy pre-packaged mixed greens or buy or grow an assortment of different salad greens like arugula, mache, dandelion, and assorted lettuces. Allow ¼ cup Parsley Dill dressing per salad. May add avocado wedges if not limiting calories to 1600/day.

Parsley Dill Salad Dressing Recipe: Makes 1 cup dressing.
¾ cup Fat Free Plain Greek Yogurt
½ cup minced flat leaf parsley – add more parsley if you prefer a
    thicker dressing
2 Tbsp. minced red onion
2 Tbsp. fresh dill or 1 tsp. dried dill
2 Tbsp. lemon juice
1 tsp. 100% maple syrup
1/8 tsp. salt
2 Tbsp. olive oil
Mix all ingredients in a blender. Blend until smooth. Refrigerate.

Nutritional analysis per serving of salad, without addition of avocado: 116 calories, 5 g. protein, .4 g. fiber, 7 g. fat, 74 mg calcium, 96 mg. sodium.

Chocolate Covered Strawberries Recipe:

Per Person:
 4 medium to large strawberries
 2 squares 85% cocoa chocolate per person (if the 85% is too intense for you then you can use a lower cocoa content, which will have more sugar, but try not to go below 70% cocoa content). I like Lindt 85% Cocoa Extra Dark Chocolate Bars, which are available at many stores and on the Internet.

Wash strawberries and gently pat dry with paper towel. Place the chocolate in a microwave safe container. Set microwave on medium setting and microwave for 10 seconds, and then stir. Microwave another 10 seconds and stir again.   Continue microwaving and stirring in 10 second intervals until melted completely. If you prefer you can melt the chocolate on low in a pan on the stove, stirring often or in a double boiler.

Dip whole strawberries in melted chocolate, holding strawberries by the stems. Place on wax paper and allow chocolate to solidify. The chocolate will solidify more quickly if you refrigerate the dipped strawberries. If you are not going to eat them right away then refrigerate. I think they are better at room temperature.

Nutritional analysis per serving: 130 calories, 3 g. protein, 4 g. fiber, 9 g. fat, 18 mg. calcium, 8 mg. sodium.

Day 2 Menu

<u>Breakfast</u>
Oatmeal with Banana and Walnuts
½ Blueberry Smoothie
Beverage of Choice

<u>Lunch</u>
Edamame Quinoa Salad
½ Blueberry Smoothie
Beverage of Choice

<u>Dinner</u>
Fish with Achiote Rub
Mashed Cauliflower
Spinach Raspberry Salad
Beverage of Choice

If restricting sodium to 1500 mg/day: May add scant 1/8 tsp. salt to food or in cooking beyond what is already in the recipes.
2300 mg/day: May add an additional generous 3/8 tsp. salt to food or in cooking.

If not restricting calories to 1600/day:
Breakfast: May have extra oatmeal with banana.
Lunch: May have extra Edamame salad and a serving of whole grain bread.
Dinner: May have a serving of whole grain bread.

<u>Recipes</u>
<u>Breakfast:</u> Oatmeal with Banana and Walnuts, ½ Blueberry Smoothie.

Oatmeal Recipe: Makes 1 serving
¼ cup steel cut oats (may substitute rolled oats if you prefer)
1 cup unsweetened almond milk
1/4 tsp. ground cinnamon, or to taste
1/8 tsp. ground ginger, or to taste
1/2 tsp. vanilla, or to taste
1 tsp. honey or maple syrup
1 banana, sliced into bite size slices
1 Tbsp. walnuts, chopped
1 Tbsp. flaxseed (optional, just adds 37 calories and has lots of
    health benefits)

Prepare oatmeal according to package directions using almond milk instead of water. Mix in cinnamon, ginger, vanilla, honey (or maple syrup), banana, walnuts and flaxseed. Once cooked to desired consistency serve immediately.

Nutritional analysis per serving: 378 calories, 10 g. protein, 10 g. fiber, 8 g. fat, 340 mg. calcium, 182 mg. sodium.

Blueberry Smoothie Recipe: Drink ½ with Breakfast and ½ with Lunch.

Per person blend all of the following ingredients in a high-speed blender until smooth:
1 ¼ cup plain nonfat Greek Yogurt (containing 300 mg calcium per 1
    cup serving. Nutrition label will say 30% of the RDA for calcium)
1 cup raw kale
½ cup frozen or fresh blueberries (may substitute another fruit for
    blueberries)
1 medium banana
1 Tbsp. flaxseed (optional, just adds 37 calories and has lots of
    health benefits)

Add additional water or ice cubes if a different consistency is desired. If you have parsley or other greens that you need to use before they go bad then add them to your smoothie – don't let them go to waste. If not limiting calories to 1600 per day you can add any additional fruits and vegetables as desired.

Nutritional analysis per Smoothie: 340 calories, 33 g. protein, 7 g. fiber, 2 g. fat, 488 mg. calcium, 146 mg. sodium.

Lunch: Edamame Quinoa Salad, other ½ of Blueberry Smoothie.

Edamame Quinoa Salad Recipe: Makes 4 servings – make enough to have again for lunch on Day 4.

1 cup red or white quinoa, rinsed
1 ¾ cup low sodium vegetable broth or stock
10 ounces edamame (shelled soybeans) - thawed if using frozen
¼ cup dried cranberries
1 cup purple grapes, cut in half
½ cup whole cashews
1 fennel bulb, trimmed and diced
¼ cup chopped fronds (wispy green leaves) from fennel
Lemon peel from 1 organic lemon

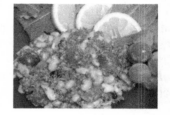

¼ cup fresh squeezed lemon juice
1 Tbsp. Dijon mustard
2 Tbsp. maple syrup
¼ cup olive oil
8 cups arugula

In medium saucepan, bring vegetable broth to a boil. Add quinoa and reduce heat to a simmer. Cover and cook 15 minutes or until broth is all absorbed. Stir half way through the cooking time. Remove from heat and let sit covered 10 minutes.

Transfer quinoa to a large bowl. Add edamame, cranberries, grape halves, cashews, fennel, fennel fronds and lemon peel.

To make dressing mix lemon juice, Dijon mustard, maple syrup and olive oil in a jar. Shake well. Carefully mix dressing into salad. Serve salad on bed of arugula – 2 cups per serving.

Nutritional Analysis per serving: 559 calories, 18 g. protein, 9 g. fiber, 28 g. fat, 170 mg calcium, 220 mg sodium.

Dinner: Fish with Achiote Rub, Mashed Cauliflower, Spinach Raspberry Salad.

Fish with Achiote Rub Recipe: Makes 4 servings – make enough for dinner and for lunch the next day.
Preheat oven to 400°F.

If you are able to get good quality fresh fish all you have to do for a great meal is simply cook or grill the fish, avoid overcooking and squeeze on some fresh lemon and ground black pepper. You may not want to cover up the taste of high quality fish with sauces or spices. If you feel the fish needs some seasoning then go with this Achiote Rub.

If you purchase already prepared Achiote paste this is a very quick and easy recipe to make. It is worth the trouble to find or make the Achiote paste for this very unique Yucatan traditional food but if you are unable to secure the Achiote or you don't want to make it from scratch then you can still rub the herbs in the recipe that are available to you on the fish and have an enjoyable entrée (as long as you are using a good quality fish and you don't overcook the fish).

Four 4 ounce fish fillets, preferably sustainable such as Arctic Char (farmed), Tilapia (Equador & US), Catfish (US) or Pacific Halibut (US).   Go to www.seafoodwatch.org   for sustainable fish purchasing guidelines.   You can also look for fish with the Marine Stewardship Council Blue eco-label in your grocery store.

You can purchase prepared achiote paste or you can make your own. If using prepared achiote paste then to 2 Tbsp. paste mix in enough orange juice to make a paste that can be rubbed on the fish. To prepare your own achiote paste:

2 Tbsp. Achiote seeds
½ tsp. black pepper
¼ tsp. ground cumin
¼ tsp. ground allspice
8 garlic cloves, peeled and minced
½ tsp. dried Mexican oregano
¼ tsp. paprika

½ tsp. sea salt
2 Tbsp. orange juice
2 Tbsp. apple cider vinegar

Use a mortar and pestle or spice grinder to grind the achiote seeds to a fine powder.   In a small bowl mix ground achiote with pepper, cumin, allspice, garlic, oregano, paprika, salt, orange juice and vinegar.   Blend to a paste.   Add additional orange juice if paste is too thick.

Rub fish fillets with Achiote paste. If you are not making the achiote sauce then just rub the spices (black pepper, cumin, allspice, garlic, oregano, paprika and the salt) on the fish.

Bake fillets on lightly oiled baking sheet at 400°F. for 10 to 12 minutes or until done (opaque but firm).   Cooking time will depend on thickness of fillets. Do not overcook. Fish continues to cook for several minutes after taken off the heat so some cooks like to remove fish from the heat source when it is just a little underdone. May also grill fish. Serve warm with fresh lime wedge.

Nutritional Analysis per serving: 124 calories, 23 g. protein, 3 g. fiber, 2 g. fat, 28 mg. calcium, 351 mg. sodium.

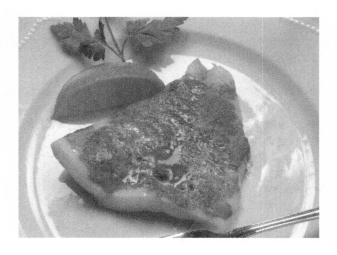

Mashed Cauliflower Recipe:

Per serving: In a saucepan cook 1 cup cauliflower with 2 garlic cloves (use more if you like) in water over medium heat until very tender. Drain cauliflower and return to saucepan. Mash cauliflower and garlic with potato masher. Add 1/8 tsp. salt, black pepper to taste and ½ tsp. olive oil. Mash until smooth.

Nutritional analysis per serving: 54 calories, 2 g. protein, 3 g. fiber, 2 g. fat, 33 mg. calcium, 322 mg. sodium.

If not restricting calories to 1600 may drizzle a little additional high quality olive oil over top of mashed cauliflower.

Spinach Raspberry Salad Recipe:

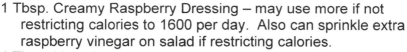

Per person:
2 cups fresh spinach
½ cup fresh raspberries
1 Tbsp. chopped walnuts
1 Tbsp. Creamy Raspberry Dressing – may use more if not restricting calories to 1600 per day. Also can sprinkle extra raspberry vinegar on salad if restricting calories.
1 Tbsp. blue cheese – optional and if not restricting calories to 1600 per day.

Mix dressing into spinach and put on salad plate. Top with raspberries, walnuts and blue cheese (optional).

Creamy Raspberry Dressing:

Put all ingredients in a jar and shake until smooth:
3 Tbsp. raspberry vinegar (balsamic or regular)
3 Tbsp. honey
1 Tbsp. plain nonfat Greek yogurt
1 tsp. Dijon mustard
¼ cup olive oil

Nutritional analysis per serving of salad without blue cheese and with 1 Tbsp. dressing: 164 calories, 4 g. protein, 6 g. fiber, 8 g. fat, 85 mg. calcium, 55 mg. sodium.

Day 3 Menu

Breakfast
2 Blueberry Muffins
½ Raspberry Smoothie
Beverage of Choice

Snack anytime during the Day
½ Raspberry Smoothie

Lunch
Fish with Achiote Rub
Apple Fennel Salad with Lemon Maple Dressing
Beverage of Choice

Dinner
Roasted Vegetables with Barley and Balsamic Reduction
Peach with Ricotta Cheese and Honey
Beverage of Choice

If restricting sodium to 1500 mg/day: May add 1/16th tsp. salt to food or in cooking beyond what is already in the recipes.
2300 mg/day: May add a generous 3/8 tsp. additional salt to food or in cooking.

If not restricting calories to 1600/day:
Breakfast: May have 1 additional muffin.
Dinner: May have a serving whole grain bread, more of the Roasted Vegetables with Barley and more Peach with Ricotta cheese.

Recipes:
Breakfast: 2 Blueberry Muffins, ½ Raspberry Smoothie.

Blueberry Muffin Recipe: Makes 12 muffins – make enough to freeze for another morning so you get 2 Breakfast from this recipe.

Preheat oven to 400° F.

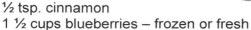

1 cup whole wheat flour
½ cup almond flour/meal
½ cup teff flour
2 tsp. baking powder
¼ tsp. salt
½ tsp. cinnamon
1 ½ cups blueberries – frozen or fresh
2 eggs
3 Tbsp. honey
2 Tbsp. molasses
½ cup almond butter
1 cup almond milk (may substitute skim milk)
½ tsp. vanilla

Mix flours, baking powder, salt and cinnamon in large bowl. Add blueberries and mix to coat blueberries with flour mixture.

In small bowl lightly beat eggs with fork. Mix in honey, molasses, almond butter, almond milk and vanilla. Add to dry ingredients and stir just until blended.

Prepare 12 muffin cups and divide batter evenly between muffin cups. Batter will come to the top of the muffin cups. Bake at 400°F. for 15 to 20 minutes or until done.

Nutrient analysis per muffin: 205 calories, 7 g. protein, 4 g. fiber, 10 g. fat, 160 mg. calcium, 159 mg. sodium.

Raspberry Smoothie Recipe: Drink ½ at Breakfast and ½ as a snack anytime during the day.

Per person blend all of the following ingredients in a high-speed blender until smooth:
1 cup plain nonfat Greek Yogurt (containing 300 mg Calcium per 1 cup serving. Nutrition label will say 30% of the RDA for Calcium)
1 cup raw spinach
1/2 cup frozen or fresh raspberries (may substitute another fruit for raspberries)
1 medium banana
1 Tbsp. flaxseed (optional, just adds 37 calories and has lots of health benefits)

Add additional water or ice cubes if a different consistency is desired. If you have parsley or other greens that you need to use before they go bad then add them to your smoothie – don't let them go to waste. If not limiting calories to 1600 per day you may add additional fruits and vegetables.

Nutritional analysis per Smoothie: 307 calories, 27 g. protein, 12 g. fiber, 1 g. fat, 366 mg. calcium, 121 mg. sodium.

Lunch: Achiote Fish (leftover from Day 2), Apple Fennel Salad.

Achiote Fish Recipe: Serve leftover fish from yesterday cold with sauce made with 2 Tbsp. Greek yogurt seasoned with 1 tsp. lime juice, 1 Tbsp. cilantro, 1/8 tsp. red pepper and 1/8 tsp. chili powder per person.

Nutritional Analysis per serving: 140 calories, 26 g. protein, 3 g. fiber, 2 g. fat, 66 mg. calcium, 363 mg. sodium.

Apple Fennel Salad Recipe:

Per person:
1 cup arugula
1 cup mixed greens
½ apple, sliced into bite size pieces
½ fennel bulb, chopped
½ cup grapes, sliced in half

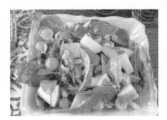

2 Tbsp. Lemon Maple Dressing
1 Tbsp. chopped walnuts

In bowl mix together arugula, greens, apple, fennel and grapes. Mix in Lemon Maple Dressing. Serve on salad plates and top with walnuts.

Lemon Maple Dressing Recipe:
Put all ingredients in a jar and shake until smooth:
2 Tbsp. 100% maple syrup
¼ cup lemon juice
1 Tbsp. Dijon mustard
¼ cup olive oil

Nutritional analysis per serving of salad: 283 calories, 4 g. protein, 6 g. fiber, 14 g. fat, 135 mg. calcium, 178 mg. sodium.

Dinner: Roasted Vegetables with Barley and Balsamic Reduction, Peach with Ricotta Cheese and Honey.

Roasted Balsamic Vegetables with Barley Recipe:
Makes 4 servings – make enough to have for dinner and for lunch later in the week.
Preheat oven to 425°F.

1 cup raw barley, cooked
3 beets with greens
1 sweet potato
2 tsp. olive oil
1 tsp. cinnamon
1/8 tsp. cayenne pepper
1/8 tsp. sea salt
½ cup Balsamic vinegar
2 garlic cloves, peeled and halved
¼ cup sunflower seeds
¼ cup dried cranberries or dried cherries, preferably unsweetened
¼ cup goat cheese

Wash beets and beet greens well.   Cut greens from beets and slice into strips. Set greens aside. Wrap beets in aluminum foil, place on a baking sheet and cook at 425° for 45 minutes or until tender all the way through (unwrap and test with fork). Allow beets to cool, and rub the skin off the beets. Cut into bite size pieces and set aside.

Wash sweet potato and cut into bite size pieces. In small bowl mix 1 tsp. olive oil, cinnamon and cayenne pepper into sweet potatoes, coating well. Roast sweet potato at 425° for 25 to 30 minutes or until tender. Set aside.

Heat 1 tsp. olive oil in large sauté pan over medium heat. Add beet greens (ok if they have a little water left on them from washing) and sauté until just wilted (don't overcook since you will need to add them to the pan again later to warm). Add salt and set aside.

Place balsamic vinegar and garlic in large sauté pan that you used to sauté greens. Cook over medium low heat until reduced by half. Remove garlic.

Add beets, sweet potatoes and beet greens to reduced balsamic vinegar in sauté pan. Cook just until vegetables are warm and greens are wilted. Mix in sunflower seeds and dried cranberries. Serve vegetable mixture over barley (may substitute other grain, brown rice or quinoa if preferred).

Top with goat cheese (2 Tbsp. per serving).

Nutritional analysis per serving: 412 calories, 14 g. pro, 14 g fiber, 175 mg calcium, 289 mg sodium.

Peach with Ricotta Cheese Recipe:

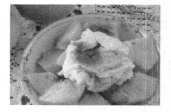

Per person:
Slice 1 peach into an individual size serving bowl. Mix ¼ cup part skim ricotta cheese with 1 tsp. honey or 100% maple syrup. Top peach with ricotta cheese mixture. Sprinkle cinnamon on top.

Nutritional analysis per serving: 165 calories, 8 g. protein, 2 g. fiber, 5 g. fat, 178 mg. calcium, 78 mg. sodium.

Day 4 Menu

Breakfast
Almond Toast
½ Cherry Smoothie
Beverage of Choice

Lunch
Edamame Quinoa Salad
½ Cherry Smoothie
Beverage of Choice

Dinner
Wheat and Barley Pilaf
Sautéed Bananas with Greek Yogurt
Beverage of Choice

If restricting sodium to 1500 mg/day: May add a scant ¼ tsp. salt to food or in cooking beyond what is already in the recipes.
2300 mg/day: May add an additional generous ½ tsp. salt to food or in cooking.

If not restricting calories to 1600/day:
Breakfast: May have 2ⁿᵈ almond toast OR 1 egg.
Lunch: May have extra Edamame salad and a serving whole grain bread.
Dinner: May have extra Wheat and Barley Pilaf, a serving whole grain bread and extra sautéed Bananas.
Snack: May have 3 cups popcorn.

Recipes
Breakfast: Almond Toast, ½ of Cherry Smoothie.

Per person:
Spread 2 Tbsp. almond butter on 1 slice toasted whole grain bread.

Nutritional Analysis for 1 Almond Toast: 250 calories, 11 g. protein, 6 g. fiber, 17 g. fat, 110 mg. calcium, 112 mg. sodium.

Cherry Smoothie recipe: To be divided to drink ½ at breakfast and ½ at lunch.

Per person blend all of the following ingredients in a high-speed blender until smooth:
½ cup unsweetened Almond Milk (Calcium calculation based on using almond milk containing 300 mg calcium per 8 ounces or 30% of the Calcium RDA. If using a product higher than 300 mg. then use only amount of Almond Milk required for 300 mg. calcium and use water for the rest of the liquid).
1 cup plain nonfat Greek Yogurt (containing 300 mg calcium per 1 cup serving. Nutrition label will say 30% of the RDA for calcium)
½ cup frozen cherries
1 cup kale
1 medium banana
1 Tbsp. ground flaxseed (optional, just adds 37 calories and has lots of health benefits)

Add additional water or ice cubes if a different consistency is desired. If you have parsley or other greens that you need to use before they go bad then add them to your smoothie – don't let them go to waste. If not limiting calories to 1600 per day you may add additional fruits and vegetables.

Nutritional Analysis per Smoothie not including flaxseed: 324 calories, 28 g. protein, 6 g. fiber, 3 g. fat, 567 mg. calcium and 212 mg. sodium.

Lunch: Edamame Salad leftover from Day 2, other 1/2 of Cherry Smoothie.

Dinner: Wheat and Barley Pilaf, Sautéed Bananas with Greek Yogurt.

Recipe for Wheat and Barley Pilaf: Makes 4 servings, ½ recipe for 2.

1 cup barley
1 tsp. olive oil for cooking barley
3 cups water or 2 ½ cups water plus ½ cup white wine
¼ tsp. sea salt
1 tsp. instant beef bouillon
¼ tsp. black pepper, or more if desired
½ tsp. garlic powder
¼ tsp. smoked paprika
¼ cup bulgur or cracked wheat
5 ounces spinach, shredded or 6 cups lightly packed spinach
½ cup sliced green onions
¼ cup flat leaf parsley, chopped
Juice of 1 lemon
1 cup cherry tomatoes, cut in half
¼ cup sunflower seeds
Optional: 4 tsp. high quality olive oil to drizzle 1 tsp. over each
    serving (if not limiting calories to 1600)

Heat olive oil over medium heat in a large skillet. Add barley and cook until golden brown, approximately 5 minutes. Mix in water, wine if using, salt, beef bouillon, pepper, garlic powder and paprika. Bring to a boil. Reduce heat to low, cover and cook for 40 minutes. Add bulgur wheat and simmer covered another 15 minutes.

Stir in spinach (add as much as will fit in the pan at one time, once it wilts add more until all the spinach is wilted and mixed in), green onions, parsley, lemon juice, tomatoes and sunflower seeds. Heat until warm and serve.

Optional: Drizzle 1 tsp. high quality olive oil over each serving if not limiting calories to 1600.

Nutritional analysis per serving: 277 calories, 11 g. protein, 12 g. fiber, 7 g. fat, 78 mg. calcium, 355 mg. sodium.

Sautéed Bananas with Greek Yogurt Recipe:

Per Person:
½ cup Greek yogurt
2 tsp. maple syrup – divided
1 banana, sliced into bite size pieces
¼ tsp. cinnamon
¼ cup orange juice
1 tsp. dark rum(optional)

Mix Greek yogurt with 1 tsp. maple syrup in a heat and freezer proof bowl. Put in freezer while preparing compote. You may want to freeze it when you start dinner so it will be even harder.

In shallow sauté pan, mix sliced banana with 1 tsp. maple syrup, cinnamon and orange juice.

Over medium heat, bring to a boil, and cook, stirring constantly, until reduced and thickened. Add dark rum, if desired. Remove yogurt from freezer. Pour banana mixture over yogurt. If desired, sprinkle top with additional cinnamon. Serve immediately.

Nutritional analysis per serving: 253 calories, 13 g. protein, 3.5 g. fiber, .5 g fat, 247 mg. calcium, 53 mg. sodium.

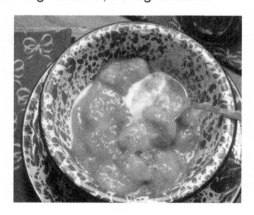

Day 5 Menu

<u>Breakfast</u>
Granola with Blueberries or Fruit of Choice
Beverage of Choice

<u>Snack anytime during the day</u>
½ Strawberry Smoothie

<u>Lunch</u>
Roasted Vegetables with Barley
½ Strawberry Smoothie
Beverage of Choice

<u>Dinner</u>
Ceviche
Baked Tortilla Chips
Beverage of Choice

If restricting sodium to 1500 mg/day: May add scant 1/4th tsp. salt to food or in cooking beyond what is already in the recipes.
2300 mg/day: May add an additional generous ½ tsp. salt to food or in cooking.

If not restricting calories to 1600/day:
Breakfast: May have extra Granola with fruit.
Lunch: May have extra Roasted Vegetables with Barley.
Dinner: May have avocado or guacamole with ceviche.

Recipes
Breakfast: ½ cup Granola with ¾ cup Non-fat Plain Greek Yogurt, ½ cup sliced blueberries and 1 tsp. honey or maple syrup if desired. May substitute another fruit for blueberries. You will need to make the Granola before the morning you plan to eat it. Store it for future use.

Granola Recipe: Makes approximately 12 cups of Granola.

Preheat oven to 300° F.

½ cup Canola Oil (preferably non GMO)
½ cup honey
½ cup maple syrup
½ cup smooth peanut butter
6 ounces prune juice
1 ½ tsp. ground cinnamon
¼ tsp. ground cloves
1 ½ tsp. ground ginger

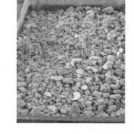

Mix the above ingredients well in a blender.

In a large bowl mix:
4 cups of rolled oats (not instant)
2 cups wheat bran (may substitute oat bran)
½ cup chopped pecans
½ cup pecan halves
1 cup sliced almonds
1 cup whole cashews

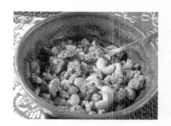

Add ingredients from blender (oil, honey etc.) to oat, bran and nut mixture. Mix until well coated.

Line 2 metal baking pans (approx.19x12x1¼ inches each) with parchment paper. Divide the granola equally between the 2 pans, spreading it in a single layer on the pans. Cook for approximately 1 hour at 300° F., stirring every 15 to 20 minutes. Once the granola is golden brown remove from the oven. Cool and store in an airtight container.

Nutritional analysis per ½ cup serving Granola with ¾ cup Greek Yogurt and ½ cup blueberries: 423 calories, 24 g. protein, 7 g. fiber, 16 g. fat, 268 mg. calcium, 75 mg. sodium.

Snack anytime during the day: ½ Strawberry Smoothie.

Strawberry Smoothie recipe: Makes 1 Smoothie. Drink ½ as a snack and ½ with Lunch.

Per person blend all of the following ingredients in a high-speed blender until smooth:
3/4 cup of unsweetened Almond Milk (Calcium calculation based on using almond milk containing 300 mg calcium per 8 ounces or 30% of the calcium RDA. If using a product higher than 300 mg. then use only amount of Almond Milk required for 300 mg. calcium and use water for the rest of the liquid).
½ cup plain nonfat Greek Yogurt (containing 300 mg calcium per 1 cup serving. Nutrition label will say 30% of the RDA for calcium)
1 cup raw kale
1 cup raw spinach
1/2 cup frozen or fresh strawberries (may substitute another fruit for strawberries)
1 medium banana
1 Tbsp. flaxseed (optional, just adds 37 calories and has lots of health benefits)

Add additional water or ice cubes if a different consistency is desired. If you have parsley or other greens that you need to use before they go bad then add them to your smoothie – don't let them go to waste. If not limiting calories to 1600 per day may add additional fruits and vegetables.

Nutritional analysis per Smoothie: 266 calories, 18 g. protein, 7 g. fiber, 4 g. fat, 523 mg. calcium, 234 mg. sodium.

Lunch: Roasted Vegetables with Barley (leftover from Day 3 dinner), ½ of Strawberry Smoothie.

Dinner: Ceviche, Baked Tortillas Chips.

Ceviche Recipe:
Serves 4 – make enough for lunch the next day as well
1 pound raw halibut, cut in ½ inch cubes (preferably Pacific halibut
    and may use frozen that has been thawed in the refrigerator)
1 cup lime juice
1 medium onion, chopped
1 jalapeno pepper, finely chopped
¼ cup chopped fresh cilantro
2 tomatoes, chopped
¼ tsp. sea salt
½ tsp. ground cumin seed
1 Tbsp. fresh oregano or 1 tsp. dried oregano
¼ tsp. black pepper or to taste
3 Tbsp. olive oil

Put fish in a medium size glass container. Cover with lime juice and refrigerate for at least 3 hours.   Drain lime juice from fish.

In medium bowl mix onion, jalapeno pepper, cilantro, tomatoes, salt, cumin, oregano, black pepper and olive oil.   Mix with fish and serve.

Nutritional analysis per serving: 252 calories, 23 g. protein, 2 g. fiber, 12 g. fat, 49 mg. calcium, 235 mg. sodium

Serve with baked tortilla chips or Flackers or Multi Grain Wasa crispbreads.

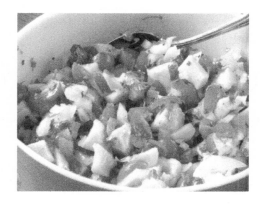

Day 6 Menu

Breakfast
**2 Banana Pancakes
1/3 of Mango Smoothie
Beverage of Choice**

Snack Anytime During the Day
2/3 Mango Smoothie

Lunch
**Ceviche
Baked Tortilla Chips
Beverage of Choice**

Dinner
**Chicken Breasts with Sautéed Mushrooms
Roasted Broccoli
Raspberry and Greens Salad
Beverage of Choice**

If restricting sodium to 1500 mg/day: Do not add salt to food or in cooking beyond what is already in the recipes and do not brine the chicken.
2300 mg/day: May add an additional ¼ tsp. salt to food or in cooking and may brine the chicken.

If not restricting calories to 1600/day:
Breakfast: May have extra pancakes.
Lunch: May have avocado or guacamole.
Dinner: May have an extra 2 ounces chicken and a serving of whole grain bread.

Recipes
Breakfast: Banana Pancakes, 1/3 of Mango Smoothie.

Banana Whole Wheat Pancakes Recipe:
Makes Eight 4-½ inch pancakes.

Pancakes
1 egg
1 cup buttermilk
2 Tbsp. canola oil
1 cup whole wheat flour
1 Tbsp. sugar
1 tsp. baking powder
½ tsp. baking soda
¼ tsp. salt
1 ripe banana, peeled and mashed
1 tsp. vanilla
½ tsp. cinnamon
¼ cup chopped pecans

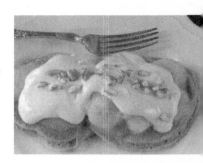

Caramelized Banana Topping
2 bananas, sliced into bite size slices
2 Tbsp. 100% maple syrup
2 cups applesauce

Cinnamon Yogurt Topping
1 cup plain non-fat Greek yogurt
2 tsp. 100% maple syrup
½ tsp. cinnamon

In medium bowl, beat egg with mixer. Add buttermilk, canola oil, whole wheat flour, sugar, baking powder, baking soda, salt, banana, vanilla and cinnamon. Mix well. Stir in pecans. Heat griddle over medium heat. For each pancake drop 1/3 cup of batter on to griddle, cooking until brown on both sides. Keep warm until ready to serve.

For topping slice 2 bananas into bite size slices. Heat 2 Tbsp. maple syrup in medium size skillet over medium heat. Cook bananas in maple syrup until just starting to soften and caramelize. Add applesauce and heat until just warm.

For yogurt topping mix yogurt with 2 tsp. maple syrup and ½ tsp. cinnamon.

To assemble pancakes, top pancakes with caramelized bananas and yogurt topping. If you can afford the extra calories add a few more pecans to top of yogurt topping.

Nutritional analysis for 2 pancakes with caramelized banana and yogurt topping: 468 calories, 15 g. protein, 8 g. fiber, 15 g. fat, 261 mg. calcium, 536 mg. sodium

(Two pancakes with ¼ cup syrup instead of topping are 554 calories & 221 mg Calcium).

Mango Smoothie recipe: To be divided to drink 1/3 at breakfast and 2/3 as a snack anytime during the day.

Per person blend all of the following ingredients in a high-speed blender until smooth:

½ cup plain nonfat Greek Yogurt (containing 300 mg calcium per 1 cup serving. Nutrition label will say 30% of the RDA for calcium)
1 ¼ cup of unsweetened Almond Milk (Calcium calculation based on using almond milk containing 300 mg calcium per 8 ounces or 30% of the calcium RDA. If using a product higher than 300 mg. then use only amount of Almond Milk required for 300 mg. calcium and use water for the rest of the liquid).
1 cup fresh or frozen mango (may substitute another fruit)
1 ½ cup kale
1 medium banana
1 Tbsp. flaxseed (optional, just adds 37 calories and has lots of health benefits)

Add additional water or ice cubes if a different consistency is desired. If you have parsley or other greens that you need to use before they go bad then add them to your smoothie – don't let them go to waste. If not limiting calories to 1600 per day may add additional fruits and vegetables as desired.

Nutritional analysis per Smoothie: 377 calories, 19 g. protein, 9 g. fiber, 6 g. fat, 698 mg. calcium, 315 mg. sodium.

Lunch: Ceviche (leftover from yesterday) and Baked Tortilla Chips.

Dinner: Chicken Breasts with sautéed mushrooms, Roasted Broccoli, Raspberry and Greens Salad.

Chicken Breasts with Sautéed Mushrooms Recipe:
Serving size is 4 ounces chicken per person.

Grill or cook chicken breasts according to your favorite method. Here are some options:
Brine: (Do not brine chicken if limiting sodium to 1500 mg. per day). 1 Tbsp. salt dissolved in 1-½ cups water for every 6 to 8 ounce chicken breast. Dissolve salt in water and submerge chicken in brine. Cover and refrigerate for at least 30 minutes or up to 1 hour. Remove chicken from brine and dry chicken on paper or lint free cloth towel. Spray or lightly brush chicken breasts with olive oil and desired seasonings. Do not use this method if limiting sodium to 1500 mg. per day. Grill, bake or sauté.

En Papillote – Preheat the oven to 375° F. Season chicken breast with olive oil and desired seasonings. Cut 15 inch squares of parchment paper (or aluminum foil). Fold square in half to make a crease in center of paper or foil. Lay chicken breast just to one side of the crease. Seal packets by loosely folding the other half of the paper or foil over the chicken. Turn up edges of paper or foil in ½ inch fold on all open edges. Smooth fold to make a sharp crease and double fold for a secure seal. Press smooth again. Bake packets on baking sheet for 15 to 25 minutes, depending on thickness of chicken, until done (160° F). Allow chicken to stand for 5 minutes prior to serving.

Overcooking chicken breasts results in dry, tough chicken. For even cooking you can pound the chicken breasts to flatten them to an even thickness.

Sautéed Mushroom topping per person:
1 cup mushrooms, sliced
1 tsp. olive oil
2 Tbsp. white wine or water
1 tsp. lemon juice
2 Tbsp. flat leaf parsley, chopped

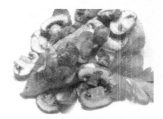

In skillet heat olive oil over medium heat. Add mushrooms and cook for 2 minutes, stirring frequently. Add water or white wine and continue to cook until water or wine has cooked off and mushrooms are tender. Mix in lemon juice and serve mushrooms on top of chicken. Sprinkle parsley over top of mushrooms.

Nutritional analysis per serving for brined chicken: 190 calories, 28 g. protein, 8 g. fat, 16 mg. calcium, 417 mg. sodium.

Roasted Broccoli Recipe

Preheat oven to 400° F.

Per person:
1 cup Broccoli, washed, dried and cut into bite size florets
1 tsp. olive oil
Black pepper to taste or use red pepper flakes
1/8 tsp. Garlic powder, if desired
Lemon juice/wedges, if desired or use red wine vinegar
Toasted almonds, if not restricting calories to 1600 per day

Place Broccoli in bowl. Add olive oil to coat broccoli (if you use your hands it will coat more evenly). Add pepper, garlic and any other desired herbs or spices – oregano, thyme, caraway seeds, coriander or tarragon work well. Evenly distribute broccoli in a single layer on a parchment lined baking pan. Bake at 400° F. for 10 to 15 minutes or until done, stirring once after 5 minutes and again as needed. Squeeze fresh lemon juice over before serving.

Nutritional analysis per serving: 70 calories, 3 g. protein, 2 g. fiber, 5 g. fat, 43 mg. calcium, 30 mg. sodium.

If not restricting calories to 1600 per day sprinkle some toasted almonds on top of the Roasted Broccoli.

Spinach Raspberry Salad Recipe:
Per person:
2 cups fresh spinach
½ cup fresh raspberries
1 Tbsp. chopped walnuts
1 Tbsp. Creamy Raspberry Dressing – may use more if not
   restricting calories to 1600 per day. Also can sprinkle extra
   raspberry vinegar on salad if restricting calories.
1 Tbsp. blue cheese – optional and if not restricting calories to 1600
   per day.

Mix dressing into spinach and put on salad plate.   Top with
raspberries, walnuts and blue cheese (optional).

Creamy Raspberry Dressing:
Put all ingredients in a jar and shake until smooth:
3 Tbsp. raspberry vinegar (balsamic or regular)
3 Tbsp. honey
1 Tbsp. plain nonfat Greek yogurt
1 tsp. Dijon mustard
¼ cup olive oil

Nutritional analysis per serving without blue cheese and with 1
Tbsp. dressing: 164 calories, 4 g. protein, 6 g. fiber, 8 g. fat, 85 mg.
calcium, 55 mg. sodium.

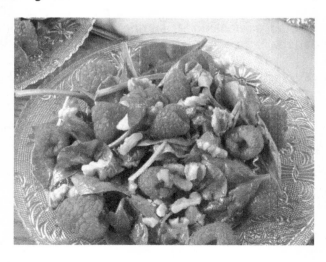

Day 7 Menu

<u>Breakfast</u>
2 Cranberry Muffins
½ Peach Smoothie
Beverage of Choice

<u>Lunch</u>
Hummus
Raw Vegetables
Whole Grain Crackers or Bread
½ Peach Smoothie
Beverage of Choice

<u>Dinner</u>
Butternut Squash Lasagna
Orange Kiwi Salad with Lemon Maple Dressing
Beverage of Choice

If restricting sodium to 1500 mg/day: Do not add salt to food or in cooking beyond what is already in the recipes.
2300 mg/day: May add a generous additional ¼ tsp. salt to food or in cooking.

If not restricting calories to 1600/day:
Breakfast: May have a 3rd muffin and an egg.
Lunch: May have additional hummus and vegetables.
Dinner: May have additional Lasagna and a serving of whole grain bread.

Recipes
Breakfast: 2 Cranberry Muffins, ½ Peach Smoothie.

Cranberry Muffin Recipe: Makes 12 muffins.
Preheat oven to 400° F.

1 cup whole wheat flour
¾ cup almond flour/meal
2 tsp. baking powder
¼ tsp. salt
1 tsp. cinnamon
½ tsp. cloves
1 Tbsp. grated orange rind, preferably from an organic orange
¼ tsp. ginger
1 ½ cups cranberries, coarsely chopped (If fresh or frozen
　　cranberries are not available substitute 1 cup plus 2 Tbsp. dried
　　cranberries)
½ cup walnuts, chopped
1 egg
1/2 cup honey
1/4 cup almond butter
3/4 cup orange juice, calcium enriched
1 tsp. vanilla

Mix flours, baking powder, salt, cinnamon, cloves, orange rind and ginger in large bowl. Add cranberries and walnuts and mix to coat with flour mixture.

In small bowl lightly beat egg with fork. Mix in honey, almond butter, orange juice and vanilla. Add to dry ingredients and stir just until blended.

Prepare 12 muffin cups and divide batter evenly between muffin cups. Batter will come to the top of the muffin cups. Bake at 400°F. for 18 to 20 minutes or until done.

Nutrient analysis per muffin: 208 calories, 6 g. protein, 4 g. fiber, 11 g. fat, 118 mg. calcium, 138 mg. sodium.

Peach Smoothie Recipe: Drink ½ with Breakfast and ½ with
   Lunch.

Per person blend all of the following ingredients in a high-speed
blender until smooth:
¾ cup plain nonfat Greek Yogurt (containing 300 mg calcium per 1
   cup serving. Nutrition label will say 30% of the RDA for calcium)
1 cup raw spinach
1 cup raw kale
1/2 cup frozen or fresh peach slices (may substitute another fruit for
   peach)
1 medium banana
1 Tbsp. flaxseed (optional, just adds 37 calories and has lots of
   health benefits)

Add additional water or ice cubes if a different consistency is
desired. If you have parsley or other greens that you need to use
before they go bad then add them to your smoothie – don't let them
go to waste. If not restricting calories to 1600 per day you may add
additional fruits and vegetables as desired.

Nutritional analysis for 1 Smoothie not including flaxseed: 291
calories, 23 g. protein, 7 g. fiber, 1 g. fat, 369 mg. calcium, 122 mg.
sodium.

Lunch: Hummus with Raw Vegetables and Crackers, ½ Peach
Smoothie.

You can make your own homemade
hummus or purchase it already made.
Try a variety of brands to determine
which one you like best.

Per person:
1/2 cup Hummus with as many raw vegetables as you like.
Try: Broccoli, cauliflower, carrot sticks, cucumbers, red pepper
slices or any other vegetable that sounds good to you.
Plus 6 whole grain crackers (I like Flackers – crackers made from
flax seeds or try Multigrain Wasa Flatbreads) or a slice of whole
grain bread.

Dinner: Butternut Squash Lasagna, Orange Kiwi Salad with Lemon Maple Dressing.

Butternut Squash Lasagna Recipe: Makes 6 generous servings – make enough for Dinner and Lunch the next day.

Preheat oven to 400° F.
4 cups peeled butternut squash, cut in to bite size cubes* or pieces
    (can use frozen)
2 tsp. smoked paprika
1 onion, chopped
1 tsp. olive oil
6 cups fresh spinach
¾ cup provolone cheese, grated
½ cup chopped flat leaf parsley
¼ tsp. pepper
1 egg
1 15-ounce carton part skim ricotta cheese
3 cups Marinara sauce (I use Rao's Homemade Marinara Sauce
    or you can make your own)
9 Lasagna noodles, cooked and well drained (draining on a lint free
    towel works well)

Coat butternut squash with paprika and spread evenly on a baking sheet (line with parchment paper if you want easy clean up). Bake for 40 minutes at 400° or until squash is tender and caramelized. If using frozen squash you may skip the cooking – just totally thaw, drain and add the paprika.

Lower oven temperature to 350°.

Heat olive oil in large pot. Sauté onions over medium heat until tender. Add spinach (it is ok if the spinach still has water clinging to it from washing) and cook until spinach wilts, about 3 to 4 minutes, stirring frequently.   Remove from pan and drain on paper or cloth towels.

Mix Provolone cheese, parsley, pepper, egg and ricotta cheese in medium bowl.
Lightly coat 8-inch square baking dish with olive oil. Spread ½ cup of marinara sauce on bottom of pan.   Arrange 3 noodles over

sauce. Spread ½ of cheese mixture over noodles. Arrange squash mixture over cheese mixture and spread ¾ cup sauce over squash. Arrange 3 noodles over sauce and spread remaining cheese mixture over the noodles. Arrange spinach onion mixture over cheese mixture and spread ¾ cup sauce over spinach onion mixture. Arrange 3 noodles over sauce and cover with 1 cup Marinara sauce. Cover pan with foil. Bake at 350° for 45 minutes or until thoroughly heated.

* To prep squash cut off top and end. Peel with vegetable peeler. Cut squash in half lengthwise and scoop out seeds. Cut squash into long slices. Cut across slices to make cubes. Google "how to cut a Butternut Squash" for some other creative ways to cut open squash.

Nutritional Analysis per serving: 459 calories, 22 g. protein, 12 g. fiber, 14 g. fat, 429 mg. calcium, 702 mg. sodium.

Orange Kiwi Salad with Maple Lemon Dressing Recipe:

Per person:
1 cup mixed greens
¼ cup shredded red cabbage
½ orange, sectioned
¼ Kiwi, sliced into bite size pieces

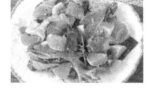

Carefully mix all salad ingredients in a bowl. Add Maple Lemon Dressing – if limiting calories to 1600 per day use 1 Tbsp. dressing per person. If not limiting calories may add sunflower seeds and avocado chunks to salad.

Maple Lemon Dressing Recipe:
Mix following ingredients together in a jar and shake until well blended:
2 Tbsp. maple syrup
¼ cup fresh lemon juice
1 Tbsp. Dijon Mustard
¼ cup olive oil

Nutritional analysis per serving with 1 Tbsp. dressing: 119 calories, 2 g. protein, 4 g. fiber, 5 g. fat, 76 mg. calcium, 52 mg. sodium.

Day 8 Menu

Breakfast
Oatmeal with Blueberries
2/3 Pineapple Smoothie
Beverage of Choice

Lunch
Butternut Squash Lasagna
1/3 Pineapple Smoothie
Apple or Fruit of Choice
Beverage of Choice

Dinner
Fish with 5 Spice Rub
Curried Cauliflower
½ Baked Sweet Potato with 1 tsp. butter
Banana Soft Serve
Beverage of Choice

If restricting sodium to 1500 mg/day: May add 1/16th tsp. salt to food or in cooking beyond what is already in the recipes.
2300 mg/day: May add an additional generous 3/8 tsp. salt to food or in cooking.

If not restricting calories to 1600/day:
Breakfast: May have more oatmeal with fruit.
Lunch: May have more Lasagna and a serving whole grain bread.
Dinner: May have a serving whole grain bread and more banana soft serve.

Recipes
Breakfast: Oatmeal with Blueberries, 2/3 Pineapple Smoothie.

Oatmeal with Blueberries and Walnuts Recipe: Makes 1 serving.

¼ cup steel cut oats (may substitute rolled oats if you prefer)
1 cup unsweetened almond milk
1/4 tsp. ground cinnamon, or to taste
1/8 tsp. ground ginger, or to taste
1/2 tsp. vanilla, or to taste
1 tsp. honey or maple syrup
1 Tbsp. flaxseed (optional, just adds 37 calories and has lots of
    health benefits)
½ cup blueberries
1 Tbsp. walnuts, chopped

Prepare oatmeal according to package directions using almond milk instead of water. Mix in cinnamon, ginger, vanilla, honey (or maple syrup) and flaxseed.   Once cooked to desired consistency add blueberries and walnuts and serve immediately.

Nutritional analysis per serving not including flaxseed: 328 calories, 10 g. protein, 9 g. fiber, 8 g. fat, 341 mg. calcium, 182 mg. sodium.

Pineapple Smoothie recipe: Drink 2/3's with Breakfast and 1/3 with Lunch.

Per person blend all of the following ingredients in a high-speed blender until smooth:
¾ cup plain nonfat Greek Yogurt (containing 300 mg. calcium per 1
    cup serving. Nutrition label will say 30% of the RDA for calcium)
1 cup raw spinach
½ cup frozen, canned or fresh pineapple (may substitute another
    fruit for pineapple)
1 medium banana
1 Tbsp. flaxseed (optional, just adds 37 calories and has lots of
    health benefits)

Add additional water or ice cubes if a different consistency is desired. If you have parsley or other greens that you need to use before they go bad then add them to your smoothie – don't let them go to waste. If not restricting calories to 1600 per day you may add additional fruits and vegetables as desired.

Nutritional analysis per serving not including flaxseed: 246 calories, 20 g. protein, 4 g. fiber, 1 g. fat, 271 mg. calcium, 97 mg. sodium.

Lunch: Butternut Squash Lasagna (leftover from last night's dinner), 1/3 pineapple Smoothie.

Dinner: Fish with 5 Spice Rub, Curried Cauliflower, ½ Baked Sweet Potato with 1 tsp. butter, Banana Soft Serve.

Fish with Five Spice Powder Rub Recipe:

If you are able to get good quality fresh fish all you have to do for a great meal is simply cook or grill the fish, avoid overcooking and squeeze on some fresh lemon and ground black pepper. You may not want to cover up the taste of high quality fish with sauces or spices. If you feel the fish needs some seasoning then go with this Five Spice Powder rub.

Preheat oven to 400° F. if not grilling fish.

Per person:
4 ounces fish, preferably sustainable such as Arctic Char (farmed),
    Tilapia (Ecuador & US), Catfish (US) or Pacific Halibut (US).
    Look for fresh, good quality fish. Go to www.seafoodwatch.org
    for the most recent sustainable fish purchasing guidelines. You
    can also look for fish with the Marine Stewardship Council Blue
    eco-label in your grocery store. The success of any fish recipe is
    greatly dependent on the quality of the fish and avoiding
    overcooking.
2 Tbsp. Five Spice Powder*
¼ cup white wine or water, if not grilling

Rub Five Spice powder on fish.

Cook fish on grill until just done. If not grilling fish place in baking dish, add white wine or water and bake uncovered at 400° for 12 to 15 minutes or until just done. Avoid overcooking which will dry the fish out. Fish continues to cook for several minutes after taken off the heat so some cooks like to remove fish from the heat source when it is just a little underdone. Serve with lime or lemon wedge.

*You can purchase Five Spice Powder or make your own. To make your own mix 1 Tbsp. ground cinnamon, ½ tsp. ground anise, ½ tsp. ground fennel seed, ½ tsp. ground black pepper and ¼ tsp. ground cloves.

Nutritional analysis per serving: 109 calories, 23 g. protein, 0 g. fiber, 2 g. fat, 11 mg. calcium, 59 mg. sodium.

Curried Cauliflower Recipe: Makes 3 servings.
3 cups cauliflower florets
¼ cup raisins
1 Tbsp. curry powder
¼ tsp. sea salt
1 cup apple juice

Mix raisins, curry powder, salt and apple juice in medium saucepan over medium heat. Add cauliflower. Bring to a simmer, cover pan and cook for 4 minutes. Remove lid and stir. Cover again and cook 4 more minutes. Remove lid and check for doneness. Once cauliflower is tender remove from heat and serve with slotted spoon, draining juice from cauliflower.

Nutritional analysis per serving: 68 calories, 3 g. protein, 4 g. fiber, .5 g. fat, 38 mg. calcium, 226 mg. sodium.

Baked Sweet Potato Recipe:
1/2 sweet potato per person if limiting calories to 1600/day. May have a whole sweet potato if not limiting calories. Scrub well and bake at 425° F. for 1 hour or until done. Pierce with fork after sweet potato has been in the oven for 30 minutes. If you have more than 1 tsp. of butter on the potato you will exceed 1600 calories for the day. I don't advocate the use of butter on a regular basis but there are certain foods that warrant butter and in my opinion a baked sweet potato is one of them.

Nutritional analysis for 1 medium baked Sweet Potato with 1 tsp. salted butter: 137 calories, 2 g. protein, 5 g. fiber, 4 g. fat, 43 mg. calcium, 75 mg. sodium.

Banana Soft Serve Recipe:

Per serving:
1 Ripe Banana, peeled and sliced into 1 inch pieces, frozen until
   solid
1 Tbsp. Almond Butter
1 Tbsp. Almond Milk
1 tsp. Maple syrup

Wrap banana slices in plastic wrap and freeze until hard. Recipe works best if bananas have been in the freezer for 2 to 3 hours. If they have frozen overnight it may take a longer to process the ice cream to the desired consistency but will still work well.

In a high speed blender or food processor (for single or small servings a small processor or blender container works better than a full size), blend frozen banana slices, almond butter, almond milk and maple syrup. It should be the texture of soft serve ice cream. Sprinkle top with cinnamon. You can eat it right away or put it in the freezer for a few minutes if you want it more solidified.

Nutrient Analysis per serving: 223 calories, 5 g. protein, 5 g. fiber, 9 g. fat, 85 mg. calcium, 14 mg. sodium.

Variations: Add a little allspice, cardamom, cloves, ginger, vanilla or nutmeg to taste. If not limiting calories to 1600 per day add a little vanilla, rum, brandy or banana liqueur. Garnish with chopped pecans, almond slices, cashews, walnuts, chocolate, coconut, dates, orange wedges, pomegranate arils, raspberries or strawberries.

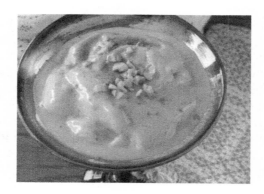

Day 9 Menu

<u>Breakfast</u>
Almond Toast with Dried Apricots
½ Strawberry Smoothie
Beverage of Choice

<u>Lunch</u>
Quinoa Raspberry Beet Salad
½ Strawberry Smoothie
Beverage of Choice

<u>Snack</u>
1 ounce Mozzarella Cheese
1 Orange or Fruit of choice

<u>Dinner</u>
Eggplant Tacos
Black Beans
Beverage of Choice

If restricting sodium to 1500 mg/day: May add 1/16th tsp. salt to food or in cooking beyond what is already in the recipes.
2300 mg/day: May add an additional generous 3/8 tsp. salt to food or in cooking.

If not restricting calories to 1600/day:
Breakfast: May have extra almond toast.
Lunch: May have extra quinoa salad and a serving whole grain bread.
Dinner: May have extra eggplant tacos and black beans plus avocado or guacamole.

Recipes
Breakfast: Almond Toast with Dried Apricots, ½ Strawberry Smoothie.

Per person:
Spread 2 Tbsp. almond butter on 1 slice toasted whole grain bread. Chop 4 Dried Apricot halves and spread evenly over the top of almond butter. If not restricting calories to 1600 sprinkle a few sliced almonds on top.

Nutritional Analysis for 1 Almond Toast with 4 dried apricot halves: 284 calories, 12 g. protein, 7 g. fiber, 17 g. fat, 118 mg. calcium, 113 mg. sodium.

Strawberry Smoothie recipe: Drink ½ at Breakfast and ½ at Lunch.

Per person blend all of the following ingredients in a high-speed blender until smooth:
¼ cup of unsweetened Almond Milk (Calcium calculation based on
    using almond milk containing 300 mg calcium per 8 ounces or
    30% of the calcium RDA. If using a product higher than 300 mg.
    then use only amount of Almond Milk required for 300 mg.
    calcium and use water for the rest of the liquid).
1 cup plain nonfat Greek Yogurt (containing 300 mg calcium per 1
    cup serving. Nutrition label will say 30% of the RDA for calcium)
1 ½ cups raw kale
1/2 cup frozen or fresh strawberries (may substitute another fruit for
    strawberries)
1 medium banana
1 Tbsp. flaxseed (optional, just adds 37 calories and has lots of
    health benefits)

Add additional water or ice cubes if a different consistency is desired. If you have parsley or other greens that you need to use before they go bad then add them to your smoothie – don't let them go to waste. If not limiting calories to 1600 per day may add additional fruits and vegetables as desired.

Nutritional analysis per Smoothie: 320 calories, 29 g. protein, 7 g. fiber, 2 g. fat, 544 mg. calcium, 181 mg. sodium.

<u>**Lunch:**</u> Quinoa Raspberry Beet Salad, ½ Strawberry Smoothie.

Quinoa Raspberry Beet Salad Recipe: Makes 4 servings – make enough to have for lunch 2 days this week.
Preheat oven to 400° F.

1 cup quinoa, rinsed
4 small beets, fresh or frozen
1 tsp. olive oil
1 1/3 cup fresh raspberries, divided
1 Tbsp. honey
¼ cup raspberry balsamic vinegar, or any balsamic vinegar will work
¼ cup walnut oil
¼ cup celery, chopped
¼ cup red onion, chopped
¼ tsp. sea salt
2 cups fresh spinach
2 cups red leaf lettuce
¼ cup roughly chopped cilantro
¼ cup walnuts, coarsely chopped
¼ cup goat cheese (can substitute feta but it will be higher in
    sodium, which you can avoid by leaving the salt out of the recipe)

Rinse quinoa well. In medium pan bring 2 cups water and quinoa to a boil. Reduce heat to low and cook covered 15 to 20 minutes, or until done and all of liquid is absorbed. (Stir quinoa half way through the cooking time). Remove from heat and let stand for 5 minutes. Then transfer quinoa to a large bowl to cool.

If using fresh beets cut off green tops, if still attached, and save for use with sautéed greens at another meal or use in a smoothie. Scrub beets well. Peel and cut beets into bite size pieces. Coat beets in olive oil. Distribute beets evenly on a parchment lined baking sheet and cook at 400° F for 15 to 20 minutes or until done.

To make dressing put 1/3 cup raspberries, honey and balsamic vinegar in a food processor bowl or blender. Process until well pureed. Add walnut oil to raspberry mixture and blend until smooth. If desired, strain to remove the raspberry seeds. They don't bother me so I leave the seeds in the dressing.

To large bowl with quinoa add celery, red onion, salt, beets, spinach, lettuce and cilantro. Gently mix dressing into salad. Serve, topping each serving with 1 Tbsp. walnuts, ½ cup raspberries and 1 Tbsp. goat cheese.

Nutrient analysis per serving: 465 calories, 12 g. protein, 9 g. fiber, 25 grams fat, 120 mg. calcium, 274 mg. sodium.

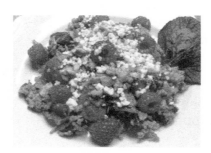

Dinner: Eggplant Tacos, Black Beans.

Eggplant Tacos Recipe: Makes 4 Tacos, 2 tacos per serving
Preheat oven to 425° F.

3 cups eggplant, cut into ½ inch or smaller bite size pieces
2 cups cherry tomatoes
1 tsp. olive oil (may use more if not limiting calories to 1600/day)
1/8 tsp. sea salt
½ tsp. chili powder (less if you prefer less spicy/hot)
¼ tsp. black pepper
4 whole wheat or whole grain flour tortillas, warmed
¼ cup chutney (can use salsa or pepper jelly instead)
4 Lime wedges

In a medium bowl, mix eggplant, tomatoes, olive oil, salt, chili powder and pepper. Evenly distribute on a parchment lined baking sheet. Roast in 425° F. oven for about 15 minutes or until eggplant is done and tomatoes are starting to pop and split.

Serve eggplant mixture in whole grain tortillas with 1 Tbsp. chutney per taco (may use more if not limiting calories to 1600 per day). Can substitute salsa or pepper jelly for chutney if you prefer. Serve with lime wedges.

Nutritional analysis for 2 tacos with chutney: 313 calories, 10 g. protein, 12 g. fiber, 4 g. fat, 57 mg. calcium, 588 mg. sodium.

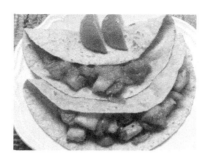

Black Beans Recipe:

Per Person:
½ cup Black Beans - I like Eden No Salt Added canned beans with BPA free lining or try Whole Foods 365 Organic No salt added beans that are packed in cartons. If you have time cook your own from dried beans, adding seasonings at beginning of cooking time.
1 Tbsp. chopped onion
1 garlic clove, minced
1/8 tsp. cumin
¼ tsp. Mexican oregano
1/8 tsp. epazote (may omit if not available)
Black pepper to taste
2 Tbsp. plain, nonfat Greek Yogurt

Mix onion, garlic, cumin, oregano, epazote and pepper into beans. If desired, mash with potato masher. Warm and serve with Greek yogurt on top. If not limiting calories to 1600/day you may cook onion and garlic over low heat in olive oil until tender.   Then add beans and spices.

Nutritional analysis per serving: 127 calories, 10 g. protein, 6 g. fiber, 1 g. fat, 98 mg. calcium, 27 mg. sodium.

Day 10 Menu

Breakfast
Ricotta English Muffin with Strawberries
1 Egg cooked any way
Beverage of Choice

Lunch
Hummus
Raw Vegetables
Whole Grain Crackers or Bread
Cherry Smoothie
Beverage of Choice

Dinner
Acorn Squash stuffed with Farro
Sautéed Mushrooms
Roasted Broccoli
Berries Romanoff
Beverage of Choice

If restricting sodium to 1500 mg/day: May add 1/16th tsp. salt to food or in cooking beyond what is already in the recipes.
2300 mg/day: May add an additional generous 3/8th tsp. salt to food or in cooking.

If not restricting calories to 1600/day:
Breakfast: May have second egg and second English Muffin with Strawberries.
Lunch: May have extra hummus and vegetables.
Dinner: May have extra squash, a serving whole grain bread and more Berries Romanoff.

Recipes
Breakfast: Ricotta English Muffin with Strawberries, 1 Egg cooked any way.

For each serving:
1 Whole grain English muffin
½ cup ricotta cheese
1 tsp. honey
4 medium strawberries, sliced

Split English muffin in half and toast if desired. Mix ricotta cheese with honey and spread evenly over 2 English muffin halves. Layer strawberries on top of cheese mixture.

Nutritional analysis per serving: 342 calories, 20 g. protein, 5 g. fiber, 11 g. fat, 520 mg. calcium, 396 mg. sodium.

Lunch: Hummus with Raw Vegetables and Crackers, Cherry Smoothie

You can make your own homemade hummus or purchase it already made. Try a variety of brands to determine which one you like best.

Per person:
1/2 cup Hummus with as many raw vegetables as you like.
Try: Broccoli, cauliflower, carrot sticks, cucumbers, red pepper slices or any other vegetable that sounds good to you.
Plus 6 whole grain crackers (I like Flackers – crackers made from flax seeds or try Multigrain Wasa Flatbreads) or a slice of whole grain bread.

Cherry Smoothie: Drink at Lunch.
Per person blend all of the following ingredients in a high-speed blender until smooth:
1/2 cup plain nonfat Greek Yogurt (containing 300 mg calcium per 1
    cup serving. Nutrition label will say 30% of the RDA for calcium)
½ cup frozen cherries
½ cup frozen beets
½ medium banana
1 Tbsp. ground flaxseed (optional, just adds 37 calories and has lots
    of health benefits)

Add additional water or ice cubes if a different consistency is desired. I like to leave this Smoothie thick and eat it with a spoon.

Nutritional Analysis per Smoothie not including flaxseed: 182 calories, 14 g. protein, 5 g. fiber, 1 g. fat, 174 mg. calcium, 102 mg. sodium.

Dinner: Acorn Squash stuffed with Farro, Sautéed Mushrooms, Roasted Broccoli, Berries Romanoff.

Acorn Squash stuffed with Farro Recipe: Makes 2 servings
Preheat oven to 400° F.

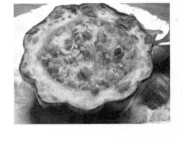

1 Tbsp. olive oil
1 Tbsp. honey
Juice of 1 lemon, preferably Meyer
1 Acorn squash
½ cup Farro, rinsed
1 ½ cups water
1/8 tsp. turmeric
1 clove garlic, minced
¼ tsp. sea salt
½ tsp. sumac berries, ground
¼ cup parmesan cheese - divided
Chopped pecans if not limiting calories to 1600 per day
Dried Cranberries, preferably unsweetened, if not limiting calories to
   1600 per day

In a small bowl combine olive oil, honey and lemon juice.

Slice Acorn Squash in half and remove seeds. Cut end off squash so it sits flat. Brush inside with some of the olive oil and lemon mixture. Bake, cut side up, at 400° F. for 20 minutes. Brush more of the olive oil and lemon mixture on the squash and bake until tender, about another 20 minutes. Reduce heat to 350°F. once squash is done and removed from oven.

While squash is baking place farro in saucepan with water. Bring to a boil, reduce heat to low and cook, covered, for 15 to 20 minutes or until done. (Or follow package directions on farro). Stir turmeric, garlic, salt, ground sumac, 2 Tbsp. parmesan cheese and remaining olive oil and lemon mixture into farro. Cook over low heat until all of liquid is absorbed.

Stuff acorn squash with farro mixture and heat at 350° for 10 to 15 minutes or until warm. Top with 1 Tbsp. parmesan cheese on each squash half.

If not restricting calories to 1600 per day may add some chopped pecans and dried cranberries to farro stuffing or to top of each squash half.

Nutritional Analysis per serving without pecans or dried cranberries: 399 calories, 13 g. protein, 8 g. fiber, 11 grams fat, 207 mg. calcium, 153 mg. sodium.

Sautéed Mushrooms Recipe:

Per person:
1 cup mushrooms, cleaned, stems trimmed, sliced
1 tsp. olive oil
1 Tbsp. White wine
1 tsp. fresh or ½ tsp. dried Thyme
1/8 tsp. black pepper, or to taste

In skillet, heat olive oil over medium high heat. Add mushrooms and cook, stirring frequently, until mushrooms release liquid. Then increase heat to high and cook, stirring frequently, until liquid from mushrooms evaporates. Reduce heat to medium and add white wine and continue to cook until mushrooms are tender and wine has evaporated. Sprinkle with thyme and pepper then serve.

Nutritional analysis per serving: 54 calories, 2 g. protein, 1 g. fiber, 5 g. fat, 2 mg. calcium, 4 mg. sodium.

Roasted Broccoli Recipe:
Preheat oven to 400° F.
Per person:

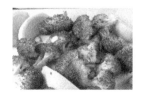

1 cup Broccoli, washed, dried and cut into bite size florets
1 tsp. olive oil
Black pepper to taste or use red pepper flakes

1/8 tsp. Garlic powder, if desired
Lemon juice/wedges, if desired or use red wine vinegar
Toasted almonds, if not restricting calories to 1600 per day

Place broccoli in bowl. Add olive oil to coat broccoli (if you use your hands it will coat more evenly). Add pepper, garlic and any other desired herbs or spices – oregano, thyme, caraway seeds, coriander or tarragon work well. Evenly distribute broccoli in a single layer on a parchment lined baking pan. Bake at 400° F. for 10 to 15 minutes or until done, stirring once after 5 minutes and again as needed. Squeeze fresh lemon juice over before serving.

Nutritional analysis per serving: 70 calories, 3 g. protein, 2 g. fiber, 5 g. fat, 43 mg. calcium, 30 mg. sodium.

If not restricting calories to 1600 per day sprinkle some toasted almonds on top of the Roasted Broccoli.

Berries Romanoff Recipe:
Per person:
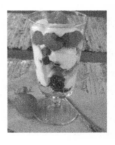
¼ cup fresh raspberries
¼ cup fresh blackberries
¼ cup fresh blueberries
¼ cup fresh strawberries
½ cup plain nonfat Greek yogurt
1 tsp. maple syrup
1 tsp. orange liquor (may substitute orange juice)
1 tsp. brandy or brandy extract (may substitute vanilla)

For each serving carefully mix berries. You can use whatever combination you want of berries if you don't want to use 4 kinds.

Mix plain nonfat Greek yogurt with maple syrup, orange liquor such as Grand Marnier or Cointreau (may substitute orange juice) and brandy or brandy extract (may substitute vanilla). Top berries with yogurt mixture or layer yogurt mixture between berries.

Nutritional analysis per serving: 160 calories, 13 g. protein, 6 g. fiber, 1 g. fat, 182 mg. calcium, 50 mg. sodium.

Day 11 Menu

Breakfast
Granola with Strawberries or Fruit of Choice
Beverage of Choice

Snack anytime during the day
½ Raspberry Smoothie

Lunch
Quinoa Raspberry Beet Salad
½ Raspberry Smoothie
Orange with 2 squares Dark Chocolate
Beverage of Choice

Dinner
Salmon with Pineapple Salsa
Sautéed Spinach
Roasted Carrots
Beverage of Choice

If restricting sodium to 1500 mg/day: May add 1/16th tsp. salt to food or in cooking beyond what is already in the recipes.
2300 mg/day: May add an additional generous 3/8 tsp. salt to food or in cooking.

If not restricting calories to 1600/day:
Breakfast: May have more Granola and fruit.
Lunch: May have more quinoa salad.
Dinner: May have 2 ounces extra salmon and a serving whole grain bread.

Recipes

Breakfast: ½ cup Granola with ¾ cup Non-fat Plain Greek Yogurt, ½ cup strawberries and 1 tsp. honey or maple syrup if desired. May substitute another fruit for strawberries.
Use the Granola recipe from Day 5.

Snack Anytime during the day: ½ Raspberry Smoothie – drink the other ½ with Lunch.

Raspberry Smoothie recipe: ½ as Snack, ½ with Lunch.

Per person blend all of the following ingredients in a high-speed blender until smooth:
1 cup of unsweetened Almond Milk (Calcium calculation based on using almond milk containing 300 mg calcium per 8 ounces or 30% of the calcium RDA. If using a product higher than 300 mg. then use only amount of Almond Milk required for 300 mg. calcium and use water for the rest of the liquid).
½ cup plain nonfat Greek Yogurt (containing 300 mg calcium per 1 cup serving. Nutrition label will say 30% of the RDA for calcium)
1 cup raw kale
1/2 cup frozen or fresh raspberries (may substitute another fruit for raspberries)
1 medium banana
1 Tbsp. flaxseed (optional, just adds 37 calories and has lots of health benefits)

Add additional water or ice cubes if a different consistency is desired. If you have parsley or other greens that you need to use before they go bad then add them to your smoothie – don't let them go to waste. If limiting calories to 1600 per day you may add additional fruits and vegetables as desired.

Nutritional analysis per Smoothie: 308 calories, 18 g. protein, 14 g. fiber, 5 g. fat, 586 mg. calcium, 255 mg. sodium.

Lunch: Quinoa Raspberry Beet Salad leftover from Day 9, ½ Raspberry Smoothie, 1 orange with 2 squares dark chocolate.

Dinner: Salmon with Pineapple Salsa, Sautéed Spinach, Roasted Carrots.

Salmon with Pineapple Salsa Recipe:
Makes 4 servings (cook enough salmon for lunch the next day)

Preheat oven to 400° F. if not grilling salmon.
1 pound raw salmon, preferably wild
½ cup white wine or water if not grilling
1 cup fresh pineapple, chopped or 1 cup canned pineapple (tidbits)
1 jalapeno pepper, finely chopped
¼ cup chopped red onion
1 tsp. finely chopped fresh ginger
½ tsp. curry powder

For salmon cook on grill until just done. Or put in baking dish, add white wine or water and bake uncovered for 12 to 15 minutes or until just done. Avoid overcooking which will dry the salmon out. Fish continues to cook for several minutes after taken off the heat so some cooks like to remove fish from the heat source when it is just a little underdone.

For salsa, in medium bowl mix pineapple, jalapeno, onion, ginger and curry powder.

Top salmon with pineapple salsa and serve.

Refrigerate 4 ounces of salmon per person for salad tomorrow and eat the other 4 ounces per person for dinner.

Nutritional analysis per serving: 212 calories, 25 g. protein, 1 g. fiber, 7 g. fat, 55 mg. calcium, 55 mg. sodium.

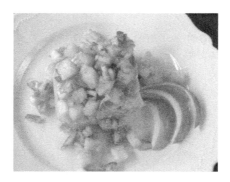

Sautéed Spinach Recipe:

For each serving/person:
1 tsp. olive oil
1 clove garlic, chopped
3 cups spinach
1/8 tsp. sea salt
Black pepper, to taste

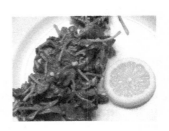

Heat 1 tsp. olive oil in skillet over medium heat. Add garlic and spinach and cook just until spinach is wilted, 3 to 4 minutes. Add salt and black pepper.

Nutritional Analysis per serving: 61 calories, 3 g. protein, 2 g. fiber, 5 g. fat, 89 mg. calcium, 362 mg. sodium.

Roasted Carrots Recipe:
Preheat oven to 400°F.

For each serving/person:
1 medium carrot, cut into bite size pieces or sticks (May use more
    carrot per serving if desired)
1 tsp. olive oil
¼ tsp. cardamom
1/8 tsp. sea salt

In a bowl coat carrot slices with olive oil. Add cardamom and salt. Evenly distribute carrots on parchment lined baking sheet and cook for 20 to 25 minutes at 400° F. or until tender. Stir half way through cooking time. Remove from oven when done.

Nutritional Analysis per serving: 65 calories, .5 g. protein, 2 g. fiber, 5 g. fat, 20 mg. calcium, 333 mg. sodium.

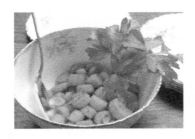

Day 12 Menu

Breakfast
Almond Toast
Greek Yogurt with Blackberries
Beverage of Choice

Snack Anytime during the Day
Mango Smoothie

Lunch
Salmon Blueberry Salad with Balsamic Dressing
Beverage of Choice

Dinner
Sweet Potato Quesadilla
Chocolate Covered Strawberries
Beverage of Choice

If restricting sodium to 1500 mg/day: May add a generous 1/8th tsp. salt to food or in cooking beyond what is already in the recipes. **2300 mg/day:** May add an additional generous ½ tsp. salt to food or in cooking.

If not restricting calories to 1600/day:
Lunch: May have avocado in Salmon salad.
Dinner: May have guacamole and extra chocolate strawberries.

Recipes:
Breakfast: Almond Toast, Greek yogurt with blackberries.

Per person:
Spread 2 Tbsp. almond butter on 1 slice toasted whole grain bread.
Mix ½ cup blackberries with ½ cup Plain Nonfat Greek Yogurt and 1
tsp. honey.

Nutritional Analysis for 1 Almond Toast: 250 calories, 11 g. protein,
6 g. fiber, 17 g. fat, 110 mg. calcium, 112 g. sodium.
Nutritional Analysis for blackberries and yogurt: 96 calories, 13 g.
protein, .4 g. fat, 4 g. fiber, 171 mg. calcium, 49 mg. sodium.

Snack anytime during the day: Mango Smoothie.

Mango Smoothie recipe: As a snack anytime during the day.

Per person blend all of the following ingredients in a high-speed
blender until smooth:
1 ¼ cup of unsweetened Almond Milk (Calcium calculation based on
   using almond milk containing 300 mg calcium per 8 ounces or
   30% of the calcium RDA. If using a product higher than 300 mg.
   then use only amount of Almond Milk required for 300 mg.
   calcium and use water for the rest of the liquid).
½ cup fresh or frozen mango (may substitute another fruit)
1 cup kale
1 medium banana
1 Tbsp. flaxseed (optional, just adds 37 calories and has lots of
   health benefits)

Add additional water or ice cubes if a different consistency is
desired. If you have parsley or other greens that you need to use
before they go bad then add them to your smoothie – don't let them
go to waste. If not limiting calories to 1600 per day may add
additional fruits and vegetables as desired.

Nutritional analysis per Smoothie: 242 calories, 6 g. protein, 7 g.
fiber, 5 g. fat, 490 mg. calcium, 253 mg. sodium.

Lunch: Salmon Blueberry Salad.

Salmon Blueberry Salad Recipe
Per person:
2 cups fresh spinach
3 Tbsp. Balsamic Dressing
½ cup fresh blueberries
1 Tbsp. sunflower seeds
4 ounces cooked salmon

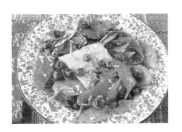

Mix dressing into spinach and put on salad plate. Top with blueberries, salmon and sunflower seeds.

Balsamic Dressing:
Put all ingredients in a jar and shake until smooth:
3 Tbsp. Balsamic vinegar (blueberry if available)
3 Tbsp. honey
1 Tbsp. plain nonfat Greek yogurt
1 tsp. Dijon mustard
¼ cup olive oil

Nutritional analysis per serving salad: 472 calories, 29 g. protein, 3 g. fiber, 22 g. fat, 114 mg. calcium, 138 mg. sodium.

Dinner: Sweet Potato Quesadilla, Chocolate covered strawberries (see Day 1 for recipe).

Sweet Potato Quesadilla Recipe: Makes 4 servings – prepare enough ingredients to make for Lunch tomorrow, too.

8 whole grain tortillas
12 ounces sweet potato, peeled and chopped
¼ cup cilantro
3 green onions, chopped
1 jalapeno pepper, chopped
1/8 tsp. sea salt
¼ tsp. cinnamon
¼ tsp. turmeric
Juice of 1 lime
1 cup cooked white beans (Navy, Cannellini) I like Eden No Salt
    Added canned beans with BPA free lining or try Whole Foods
    365 Organic No salt added beans that are packed in cartons. If

you have time cook your own from dried beans.
1 cup grated Monterrey Jack Cheese

In a medium saucepan cook sweet potato with water until tender. Remove from heat, drain well, and return to saucepan and mash. If you prefer, roast the sweet potato at 400° until tender instead – I think the flavor is better when roasted. Or you can bake the sweet potato at 400° until done and scoop out the flesh.

Mix cinnamon, turmeric, and lime juice into cooked sweet potato.

Drain beans well. In a medium bowl combine beans with cilantro, green onion, jalapeno pepper, and sea salt.

For each of 4 flour tortillas spread ¼ of sweet potato mixture over a tortilla then ¼ of bean mixture and ¼ cup cheese. Top with remaining 4 tortillas.

Heat grill pan or large non-stick skillet over medium high heat. Cook quesadillas for about 3 minutes or until lightly browned then turn and brown other side. Remove from pan and cut each quesadilla into 4 wedges. If not restricting calories to 1600 per day serve with guacamole or sliced avocado.

Guacamole Recipe
1 ripe avocado
1 tsp. lime juice
1 green onion, chopped
1 Tbsp. cilantro, chopped
¼ small tomato, chopped
1/8 tsp. sea salt
black pepper to taste
chopped jalapeno to taste (optional)

Cut avocados in half working around seed. Remove seed. Scoop out avocado from the peel, and put in a mixing bow. Mash avocado with fork and mix in lime juice, green onion, cilantro, tomato, sea salt black pepper and jalapeno pepper, if desired. Adjust seasonings to taste. Serve immediately.
Nutritional analysis per serving/1 quesadilla without guacamole or avocado: 433 calories, 19 g. protein, 13 g. fiber, 10 g. fat, 296 mg. calcium, 520 mg. sodium.

Day 13 Menu

Breakfast
Arugula Omelet
Whole Grain Toast with Jam
½ Peach Smoothie
Beverage of Choice

Lunch
Sweet Potato Quesadilla
Blueberry "Not Really Ice Cream"
Beverage of Choice

Snack anytime during the day
½ Peach Smoothie

Dinner
Pork Tenderloin in Cherry Sauce
Rosemary Potatoes
Green Beans with Artichokes
1 cup Watermelon or Fruit of Choice
Beverage of Choice

If restricting sodium to 1500 mg/day: Do not add salt to food or in cooking beyond what is already in the recipes.
2300 mg/day: May add an additional 3/8 tsp. salt to food or in cooking.

If not restricting calories to 1600/day:
Breakfast: May have a larger omelet and whole grain biscuit instead of toast.
Lunch: May have avocado or guacamole and more Blueberry "Ice Cream".
Dinner: May have extra 2 ounces of pork.

Recipes: Arugula Omelet, 1 slice Whole Grain Toast with Jam (preferably 100% fruit jam), ½ Peach Smoothie.

Arugula Omelet Recipe:

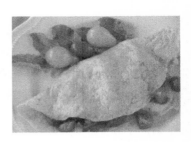

Make each omelet with:
1 tsp. olive oil - divided
2 cups arugula
2 eggs (can substitute 4 egg whites
   or 1 whole egg and 2 egg whites)
1/16th tsp. sea salt
Black pepper to taste
½ cup tomato, chopped

Heat ½ tsp. olive oil over medium heat in skillet. Add arugula to skillet and cook until just wilted. Remove arugula from pan and drain on a paper towel. Whisk eggs with salt and pepper in small bowl. Heat remaining ½ tsp. olive oil in skillet over low heat. Add eggs and prepare omelet, adding arugula and tomato just as omelet sets. Fold omelet over and serve.

Nutritional analysis for 1 omelet: 166 calories, 14 g. protein, 2 g. fiber, 10 g. fat, 128 mg. calcium, 302 mg. sodium.

Peach Smoothie Recipe: Have ½ with Breakfast and ½ as a snack anytime during the day.

Per person blend all of the following ingredients in a high-speed blender until smooth:
1 cup of unsweetened Almond Milk (Calcium calculation based on
   using almond milk containing 300 mg calcium per 8 ounces or
   30% of the calcium RDA. If using a product higher than 300 mg.
   then use only amount of Almond Milk required for 300 mg.
   calcium and use water for the rest of the liquid).
¼ cup plain nonfat Greek Yogurt (containing 300 mg calcium per 1
   cup serving. Nutrition label will say 30% of the RDA for calcium)
1 cup raw kale
1/2 cup frozen or fresh peach slices (may substitute another fruit for
   peach)
1 medium banana
1 Tbsp. flaxseed (optional, just adds 37 calories and has lots of
   health benefits)

Add additional water or ice cubes if a different consistency is desired. If you have parsley or other greens that you need to use before they go bad then add them to your smoothie – don't let them go to waste. If not restricting calories to 1600 per day you may add additional fruits and vegetables as desired.

Nutritional analysis for 1 Smoothie not including flaxseed: 259 calories, 12 g. protein, 7 g. fiber, 4 g. fat, 489 mg. calcium, 230 mg. sodium.

Lunch: Sweet Potato Quesadilla (recipe from yesterday), Blueberry "Not really ice cream".

Blueberry "Not Really Ice Cream" Recipe:

For each serving combine 1 cup frozen blueberries, ¼ cup plain, nonfat Greek yogurt and 2 tsp. maple syrup in a food processor or blender. Blend until smooth. For small serving sizes a small blender container or food processor bowl works best. Serve immediately or if you want it more frozen put in freezer until desired consistency.

Nutritional analysis per serving: 146 calories, 6 g. protein, 4 g. fiber, 1 g. fat, 96 mg. calcium, 27 mg sodium.

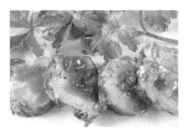

Dinner: Pork Tenderloin in Cherry Sauce, Rosemary Potatoes, Green Beans with Artichokes, 1 cup Watermelon or Fruit of Choice.

Pork Tenderloin in Cherry Sauce Recipe:
Make 4 servings (make enough for lunch the next day).
Preheat oven to 425 F. if not grilling pork.

1 (1#) Pork Tenderloin
½ tsp. ground allspice
1/8 tsp. black pepper
1/8 tsp. sea salt
½ cup Cherry preserves
    (preferably a 100% fruit version)
1 Tbsp. Brandy (optional)
1 tsp. olive oil if not grilling

In small bowl mix allspice, pepper and salt. Rub mixture evenly over pork.

In another small bowl mix cherry preserves and brandy. Brush cherry mixture over pork.

To grill sear the tenderloin on the hottest part of the grill for about 2 minutes each side. Then cook over indirect heat for 10 to 15 more minutes (not turning) until meat thermometer inserted into thickest part registers 160° F. being careful to not overcook. Remove from grill, tent with foil and let rest 5 minutes prior to serving.

To pan roast preheat oven to 400° F. Heat 1 tsp. olive oil in skillet over medium high heat. Cook pork in skillet until all sides are browned, about 2 to 3 minutes per side. Place pork on foil lined or lightly oiled baking pan. Bake at 425° F., basting once with cherry sauce, for 15 minutes or until meat thermometer inserted into thickest part registers 160° F. Remove from oven and baste with sauce again. Tent pork with foil and let rest 5 minutes prior to serving.

Cut in to medallions and serve with remaining sauce.

Nutritional Analysis including 1 tsp. olive oil: 283 calories, 30 g. protein, .4 g. fiber, 6 g. fat, 15 mg. calcium, 149 mg. sodium.

Rosemary Potatoes Recipe:
Preheat oven to 425° F.

Per person:
5 new potatoes or fingerling potatoes (between 2-1/2 & 3 ounces),
    cut into bite size wedges
1 tsp. olive oil
1-1/2 tsp. fresh Rosemary, chopped
1 tsp. flat leaf parsley, chopped
1/8 tsp. garlic powder
1/8 tsp. black pepper

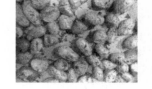

In bowl coat potatoes with olive oil. Add rosemary, parsley, garlic powder and pepper.

Evenly distribute potatoes on parchment lined baking sheet. Bake at 425° for 30 to 40 minutes or until potatoes are tender.

Nutritional analysis per serving: 106 calories, 1 g. protein, 1 g. fiber, 5 g. fat, 6 mg. calcium, 4 mg. sodium.

Roasted Green Beans with Artichokes Recipe:
Preheat oven to 425°F.

For each serving/person:
1 cup green beans, stem ends cut off
1 tsp. olive oil
Black pepper to taste
2 Artichoke hearts, sliced into bite size pieces – low sodium

Place green beans in bowl. Add olive oil to coat green beans (if you use your hands it will coat more evenly). Add black pepper. Evenly distribute green beans in a single layer on a parchment lined baking pan. Bake at 425° F. for 8 to 10 minutes or until done, stirring once after 5 minutes. Add artichoke heart slices just before serving.

Alternative Cooking method: If you have good quality green beans (fresh from Farmer's Market or your own garden) or haricots verts then you can simply boil them or sauté them until done and add seasonings. When standard grocery store green beans are all that is available to you then roasting is often a better preparation method.

Nutritional Analysis per serving: 86 calories, 2 g. protein, 2 g. fiber, 5 g. fat, 38 mg. calcium, 66 mg. sodium.

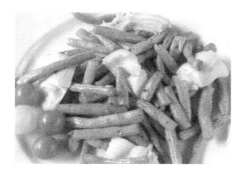

Day 14 Menu

Breakfast
2 Apricot Quinoa Muffins
2/3 of Blueberry Smoothie
Beverage of Choice

Lunch
Pork Tenderloin Cherry Salad
Beverage of Choice

Dinner
Pineapple Tomato Pizza
Spinach Kiwi Salad
1/3 Blueberry Smoothie
Beverage of Choice

If restricting sodium to 1500 mg/day: Do not add salt to food or in cooking beyond what is already in the recipes.
2300 mg/day: May add an additional 3/8 tsp. salt to food or in cooking.

If not restricting calories to 1600/day:
Breakfast: May have third muffin and 1 egg.
Lunch: May have extra pork tenderloin salad and a serving of whole grain bread.
Dinner: May add avocado to Spinach Kiwi salad.

Recipes:
Breakfast: 2 Apricot Quinoa Muffins, 2/3 of Blueberry Smoothie.

Apricot Quinoa Muffins Recipe: Makes 12 muffins – make and freeze enough for Breakfast on Day 18, too.
Preheat oven to 350° F.

½ cup uncooked quinoa, rinsed
½ cup orange juice
½ cup water
1 cup almond milk
1 Tbsp. ground flaxseed
¼ cup canola oil
¼ cup honey
¼ tsp. almond extract
1 ¼ cups whole wheat pastry flour (may substitute regular whole
    wheat flour)
¼ cup almond meal/flour
1 ½ tsp. baking powder
½ tsp. salt
½ tsp. ground cinnamon
½ tsp. ground cardamom
½ cup dried apricots, preferably unsulphured - chopped
¼ cup sliced almonds

Preheat oven to 350°. Prepare 12 cup muffin pan.

In medium saucepan mix quinoa, orange juice and water. Bring to a boil, then reduce to a simmer. Cover and cook about 15 minutes, uncovering and stirring at 8 minutes. Quinoa is done when it appears soft and translucent and the germ ring will be visible along the outside edge of the seed. Let the quinoa rest, covered for 10 minutes, before fluffing. Just use 1 ¼ cups of the cooked quinoa in the muffins – you may have a little quinoa leftover.

In medium bowl mix almond milk and flax seed. Let stand for 1 minute then add canola oil, honey and almond extract

In separate large bowl mix whole wheat pastry flour, almond meal, baking powder, salt, cinnamon, and cardamom. Add apricots, combining so that apricots are evenly distributed and well coated with dry flour mixture.   Mix in almond milk, flax seed mixture and almonds. Add 1 ¼ cups cooked quinoa.   Stir just until blended.

Divide batter up in to 12 muffin tins. Muffin tins will be filled to the top.

Bake at 350° for 20 to 25 minutes or until toothpick inserted in center of muffins comes out clean and tops spring back when lightly touched.   If baking in paper muffin cups remove from pan immediately and cool on wire cooling rack. If not using paper muffin cups let cool 5 minutes in pan and then remove and put on wire cooling rack. Freeze leftovers for another morning.

Nutrient value for 1 muffin: 175 calories, 4 g. protein, 3 g. fiber, 8 g. fat, 101 mg. calcium, 176 mg. sodium.

Blueberry Smoothie Recipe: Drink 2/3 as Breakfast and 1/3 at Dinner.

Per person blend all of the following ingredients in a high-speed blender until smooth:

½ cup of unsweetened Almond Milk (Calcium calculation based on using almond milk containing 300 mg calcium per 8 ounces or 30% of the calcium RDA. If using a product higher than 300 mg. then use only amount of Almond Milk required for 300 mg. calcium and use water for the rest of the liquid).

3/4 cup plain nonfat Greek Yogurt (containing 300 mg calcium per 1 cup serving. Nutrition label will say 30% of the RDA for calcium)

1 cup raw kale

1 cup raw spinach

½ cup frozen or fresh blueberries (may substitute another fruit for blueberries)

1 medium banana

1 Tbsp. flaxseed (optional, just adds 37 calories and has lots of health benefits)

Add additional water or ice cubes if a different consistency is desired. If you have parsley or other greens that you need to use before they go bad then add them to your smoothie – don't let them go to waste. If you are not restricting calories to 1600 per day then may add additional fruits and vegetables as desired.

Nutritional analysis per Smoothie: 302 calories, 23 g. protein, 8 g. fiber, 3 g. fat, 517 mg. calcium, 212 mg. sodium.

Lunch: Pork Tenderloin Cherry Salad.

Pork Tenderloin Cherry Salad Recipe:

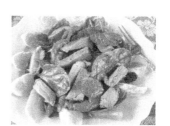

Per person:
2 tsp. apple cider vinegar
2 tsp. olive oil
2 tsp. maple syrup
1 tsp. Dijon mustard
2 cups spinach
1/4 of fennel bulb, chopped into small bite size pieces
1 Tbsp. dried cherries, chopped
1 small, sectioned orange
3 ounces pork tenderloin (cooked)

To make dressing mix vinegar, olive oil, maple syrup and Dijon mustard in jar and shake until well blended.

In bowl combine spinach and fennel with dressing. Mix in dried cherries. Arrange spinach mixture on plate and top with orange sections and pork tenderloin.

Nutritional analysis per serving: 374 calories, 25 g. protein, 6 g. fiber, 14 g. fat, 136 mg. calcium, 272 mg. sodium

Dinner: Pineapple Tomato Pizza, Spinach Kiwi Salad, 1/3 Blueberry Smoothie

Pineapple Tomato Pizza Recipe: Make enough to have for dinner and Lunch the next day.

You can make your own whole grain crust or try one of the pre-made whole grain pizza crusts now available at many grocery stores. Check out Brooklyn 100% Whole Wheat Pizza Dough in the Frozen food section. Pillsbury Artisan Pizza Crust with whole grain in the refrigerator section of the grocery store and IL Fornaio Wheat Pizza Dough in the Frozen food section aren't 100% whole grain options but do contain some whole wheat flour. If you use a pre-made pizza crust and grill the pizza this can be a fairly easy and quick meal.

Pizza Crust – makes two 12" Pizza crust:
(Freeze one crust or finished pizza for another meal if you only need one for this meal)

1 envelope dry yeast
1 cup plus 3 Tbsp. warm water (105°F to 115°F)
1 tsp. honey
1¼ cups bread flour
1¼ cups whole-wheat flour
1 Tbsp. olive oil
¾ tsp. sea salt

In small bowl sprinkle yeast over warm water. Stir in honey. Let stand until foamy.

You can mix the ingredients by hand but a food processor works better. In food processor work bowl using steel knife attachment combine bread flour, whole-wheat flour, oil and salt. With machine running add yeast mixture through feed tube and process 30 seconds. If dough sticks to bowl add more bread flour through feed tube 1 Tbsp. at a time, allowing flour to incorporate before adding additional flour if needed. If dough is dry add water through feed tube 1 tsp. at a time, allowing water to incorporate in to dough before adding additional water. Process dough until smooth and elastic, about 1 minute.

Transfer dough to large oiled bowl, turning to coat entire dough surface. Cover bowl with plastic wrap and lint free towel. Let dough rise in warm place until doubled in volume, about 1 hour. It also works well to make the dough one or 2 days ahead and refrigerate it rather than allowing it to rise at room temperature.

Punch down dough. Oil bottom of pizza pans with olive oil or use a pizza stone. Roll out dough in circles and fit to pizza pan or slide on to pizza stone. If you have chosen to refrigerate the dough instead of allowing it to rise at room temperature then remove from refrigerator when ready to use, roll and fit in to pizza pans or on to stone.

Preheat oven to 500°F. If you use a pizza stone Cook's Illustrated recommends preheating the stone for an hour at 500°F before baking Pizza on the stone. Cook's test kitchen found 30 to 45 minutes was not enough and that an hour produces the best crisp well browned crust. Cook's also recommends using an inverted baking sheet if you don't have a pizza stone and you only need to preheat it for 30 minutes since it has less mass than a stone.

If you are going to grill the pizza instead of cooking in oven see below. (I think this is the best and easiest way to prepare pizza)

Topping for 1 Pizza – double for 2:
2 cups cherry tomatoes
1/2 tsp. olive oil
1/8 tsp. cayenne pepper
2 cups pineapple bite size chunks
¼ cup red onion, chopped
¼ cup fresh cilantro
3 ounces mozzarella cheese

Heat oven heat to 400° F.
In medium bowl, mix cherry tomatoes with ½ tsp. olive oil and cayenne pepper. Evenly distribute on a baking pan. Bake at 400° for 15 to 18 minutes or until tomatoes pop open. Set aside until ready to assemble pizza.

In medium bowl, mix pineapple, red onion and cilantro.

Assembly:
If grilling pizza then see below to cook crust **before** adding tomatoes, pineapple and cheese. If grilling don't add tomatoes, pineapple or cheese to pizza until you have cooked crust on grill. If cooking in oven then put tomatoes, pineapple and cheese on before cooking crust.

To assemble pizza, distribute mozzarella cheese over pizza. Add pineapple mixture. Top with cherry tomatoes.

Bake at 500°F until crust is well browned and cheese is bubbly and beginning to brown, about 10 minutes. Rotate pizza half way through cooking time. Let pizza cool 5 minutes before cutting and serving.

Grilling directions: Roll dough out - a less than perfect rectangle is fine as you don't have to worry with getting it in a perfect round to fit on the Pizza pan. Coat one side with olive oil and take it to the grill. While walking it to the grill I stretch it a little more then place the oiled side on the grill. It bubbles up and cooks in 2 to 3 minutes on a hot grill, will take a little longer on a medium grill. Brush oil on the top or up side and flip it over to cook for just another minute or until done. The crust cooks quickly on a hot grill. Remove the crust from the grill and place it on a piece of heavy duty aluminum foil. Add your toppings and put it back on the grill, cover with grill lid and cook until cheese is melted.

Slice each pizza into 6 slices. Serving Size is 2 slices.

Nutritional analysis for 2 slices pizza: 373 calories, 16 g. protein, 5 g. fiber, 9 g. fat, 267 mg. calcium, 477 mg. sodium.

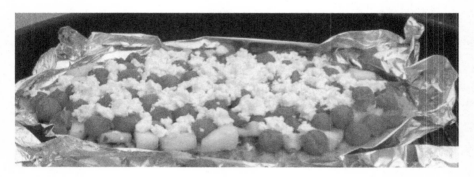

Spinach Kiwi Salad Recipe:

Per Person:
2 cups raw spinach
½ grapefruit, separated into sections
1 kiwi, cut into bite size slices
2 Tbsp. Lemon maple dressing
Avocado chunks, if not restricting calories to 1600/day
Sunflower seeds, if not restricting calories to 1600/day
To make dressing put the following ingredients in a jar and shake well:

2 Tbsp. 100% Maple syrup
¼ cup lemon juice

1 Tbsp. Dijon Mustard
¼ cup olive oil

To assemble salad mix spinach with Lemon Maple dressing. Top salad with grapefruit sections and kiwi slices. Add avocado chunks and sunflower seeds if not restricting calories to 1600 per day.

Nutritional analysis per serving without avocado and sunflower seeds: 203 calories, 3 g. protein, 4 g. fiber, 9 g. fat, 105 mg. calcium, 110 mg. sodium.

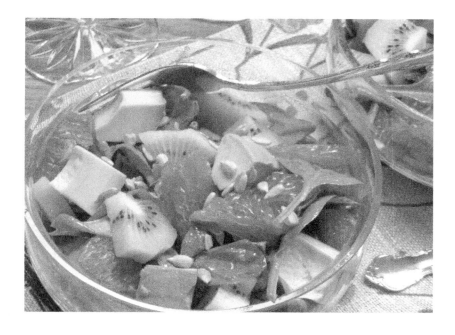

Day 15 Menu

Breakfast
Oatmeal with Dried Apricots and Raisins
½ Raspberry Smoothie
Beverage of Choice

Lunch
Pineapple Tomato Pizza
½ Raspberry Smoothie
Beverage of Choice

Dinner
Whole Grain Pasta with Arugula and Mushrooms
Beverage of Choice

If restricting sodium to 1500 mg/day: May add scant 1/8 tsp. salt to food or in cooking beyond what is already in the recipes.
2300 mg/day: May add an additional generous 3/8 tsp. salt to food or in cooking.

If not restricting calories to 1600/day:
Breakfast: May have more oatmeal and fruit.
Lunch: May have an extra slice of pizza.
Dinner: May have more pasta and a serving of whole grain bread.

Recipes
Breakfast: Steel Cut Oatmeal with Dried Apricots and Raisins, ½ of Raspberry Smoothie.

Oatmeal recipe: Makes 1 serving.

Makes 1 serving.

¼ cup steel cut oats (may substitute rolled oats if you prefer)
1 cup unsweetened almond milk
1/4 tsp. ground cinnamon, or to taste
1/8 tsp. ground ginger, or to taste
1/2 tsp. vanilla, or to taste
1 Tbsp. raisins
4 dried apricots, chopped
1 tsp. honey or maple syrup
1 Tbsp. walnuts, chopped
1 Tbsp. flaxseed (optional, just adds 37 calories and has lots of
    health benefits)

Prepare oatmeal according to package directions using almond milk instead of water. Mix in cinnamon, ginger, vanilla, raisins, apricots, honey (or maple syrup), walnuts and flaxseed. Once cooked to desired consistency serve immediately. May substitute other dried fruit such as dried cherries, dried cranberries or dried plums/prunes. May substitute other nuts or seeds for walnuts. If not restricting calories to 1600 per day may have more dried fruit and nuts than what is specified in recipe.

Nutritional analysis per serving not including flaxseed: 349 calories, 10 g. protein, 8 g. fiber, 8 g. fat, 347 mg. calcium, 183 mg. sodium.

Raspberry Smoothie recipe: To be divided to drink ½ at Breakfast and ½ at Lunch.

Per person blend all of the following ingredients in a high-speed blender until smooth:
1 cup plain nonfat Greek Yogurt (containing 300 mg calcium per 1
    cup serving. Nutrition label will say 30% of the RDA for calcium)
1 cup raw spinach
1/2 cup frozen or fresh raspberries (may substitute another fruit for

  raspberries)
1 medium banana
1 Tbsp. flaxseed (optional, just adds 37 calories and has lots of
  health benefits)

Add additional water or ice cubes if a different consistency is
desired. If you have parsley or other greens that you need to use
before they go bad then add them to your smoothie – don't let them
go to waste. If not limiting calories to 1600 per day you may add
additional fruits and vegetables.

Nutritional analysis per Smoothie: 307 calories, 27 g. protein, 12 g.
fiber, 1 g. fat, 366 mg. calcium, 121 mg. sodium.

Lunch: 2 slices Pineapple Tomato Pizza leftover from yesterday,
½ Raspberry Smoothie.

Dinner: Whole Grain Pasta with Arugula and Mushrooms

Whole Grain Pasta with Arugula and Mushrooms Recipe:

Per Person:
1 tsp. olive oil
1 garlic clove, finely chopped
¼ cup red bell pepper, chopped
½ tsp. dried oregano
1 cup sliced mushrooms
¼ cup white wine (may substitute water)
2 cups arugula
1 cup cherry tomatoes, cut in half
¾ cup Navy beans, drained (I like Eden No Salt Added canned
    beans with BPA free lining or try Whole Foods 365 Organic No
    salt added beans that are packed in cartons. If you have time
    cook your own from dried beans).
1/4 tsp. sea salt
2 Tbsp. flat leaf parsley, chopped
2/3 cup dry whole wheat penne or other whole grain pasta cooked
    according to package directions and drained
2 Tbsp. grated Parmesan cheese – divided in half
1 Tbsp. pine nuts, toasted
Fresh lemon juice to taste

To make vegetable sauce, heat olive oil in large skillet over medium heat. Add garlic, red bell pepper, oregano and mushrooms. Stirring frequently, cook for 1 minute. Add white wine (or water) to skillet. Cook until red bell pepper and mushrooms are just tender, stirring frequently. Add cherry tomatoes, navy beans and salt to skillet. Simmer over medium heat until liquid is reduced and sauce thickens. Then mix in arugula and parsley, stirring until arugula is just wilted.

Stir 1 Tbsp. Parmesan cheese into cooked, warm pasta. Serve vegetable sauce over pasta. Top with remaining 1 Tbsp. Parmesan cheese and pine nuts. Serve with lemon wedges and add lemon juice to taste. If you can afford the extra calories drizzle a little high quality olive oil over the pasta.

Nutritional analysis per serving without additional olive oil: 575 calories, 28 g. protein, 20 g. fiber, 15 g. fat, 488 mg. calcium, 494 mg. sodium.

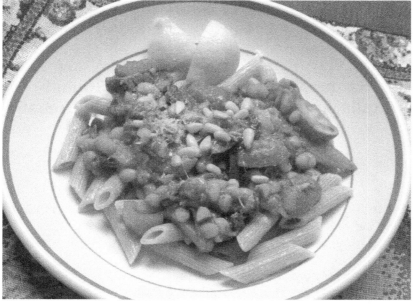

Day 16 Menu

<u>Breakfast</u>
Granola with Blackberries
Beverage of Choice

<u>Lunch</u>
Kale and Red Cabbage Salad
½ cup Raspberries
2 squares 85% dark chocolate
Beverage of Choice

<u>Snack anytime during the day</u>
Cherry Smoothie

<u>Dinner</u>
Blackened Fish
Sautéed Yellow and Zucchini Squash
Arugula Apricot Salad with Balsamic Dressing
Beverage of Choice

If restricting sodium to 1500 mg/day: Do not add salt to food or in cooking beyond what is already in the recipes.
2300 mg./day: May add additional 3/8 tsp. salt to food or in cooking.

If not restricting calories to 1600/day:
Breakfast: May have more Granola and fruit.
Lunch: May have more salad, avocado on salad and a serving whole grain bread.
Dinner: May have an additional 2 ounces fish, avocado and extra tablespoon cheese and almonds on salad and a serving of whole grain bread.

Recipes:
Breakfast: ½ cup Granola with ¾ cup Non-fat Plain Greek Yogurt, ½ cup sliced blackberries and 1 tsp. honey or maple syrup, if desired. May substitute another fruit for blackberries. Granola recipe is on Day 5.

Lunch: Kale and Red Cabbage Salad, ½ cup Raspberries, 2 squares 85% dark chocolate.

Kale and Red Cabbage Salad Recipe: Makes 4 servings – half recipe for 2 servings.

Dressing:
1 cup Navy Beans, drained – if using canned reserve the liquid (I like Eden No Salt Added canned beans with BPA free lining or try Whole Foods 365 Organic No salt added beans that are packed in cartons. If you have time cook beans from dried beans).
2 Tbsp. Tahini
2 Tbsp. Dijon Mustard
1 Tbsp. 100% maple syrup
Juice and zest of 1 Lemon
¼ cup liquid drained from Navy beans, or water if not using canned beans

Combine all ingredients in a blender and process until smooth. Add more water if needed.

Salad:
6 cups kale, shredded
2 cups red cabbage, shredded
1 cup shredded or grated carrots
3 cups Garbanzo beans, cooked – canned or made from dried beans
¼ cup sunflower seeds
Avocado chunks – if not limiting calories to 1600/day

Mix kale, red cabbage, carrots and garbanzo beans in bowl. Mix in dressing or pour dressing over top of salad once on plate. Top with sunflower seeds. May also add avocado chunks to salad if not limiting calories to 1600 per day.

Nutritional analysis per serving of salad: 248 calories, 12 g. protein, 9 g. fiber, 10 g. fat, 260 mg. calcium, 266 mg. sodium.

Snack anytime during the day: Cherry Smoothie.

Cherry Smoothie Recipe:

Per person blend all of the following ingredients in a high-speed blender until smooth:
1 cup of unsweetened Almond Milk (Calcium calculation based on using almond milk containing 300 mg calcium per 8 ounces or 30% of the calcium RDA. If using a product higher than 300 mg. then use only amount of Almond Milk required for 300 mg. calcium and use water for the rest of the liquid).
¼ cup plain nonfat Greek Yogurt (containing 300 mg calcium per 1 cup serving. Nutrition label will say 30% of the RDA for calcium)
1 cup raw kale
1/2 cup frozen cherries (may substitute another fruit for cherries)
1 medium banana
1 Tbsp. flaxseed (optional, just adds 37 calories and has lots of health benefits)

Add additional water or ice cubes if a different consistency is desired. If you have parsley or other greens that you need to use before they go bad then add them to your smoothie – don't let them go to waste. If not limiting calories to 1600 per day may add additional fruits and vegetables to Smoothie as desired.

Nutritional analysis per Smoothie: 246 calories, 12 g. protein, 7 g. fiber, 4 g. fat, 492 mg. calcium, 231 mg. sodium.

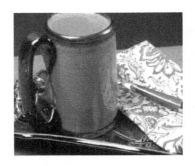

Dinner: Blackened Fish, Sautéed Yellow and Zucchini Squash, Arugula Apricot Salad with Balsamic Dressing.

Blackened Fish Recipe:

Per person:
4 ounces fish filets preferably sustainable such as Arctic Char
    (farmed), Tilapia (Ecuador & US), Catfish (US) or Pacific Halibut
    (US). Go to www.seafoodwatch.org for sustainable fish
    purchasing guidelines. You can also look for fish with the
    Marine Stewardship Council Blue eco-label in your grocery store.
1 tsp. olive oil
¼ tsp. garlic powder
½ tsp. onion powder
1/8 tsp. cayenne pepper (use less if you want less heat)
½ tsp. paprika – may use half regular paprika and half smoked or all
    regular
1/8 tsp. sea salt
¼ tsp. black pepper
¼ tsp. thyme
1/8 tsp. ground cumin
Lemon wedge

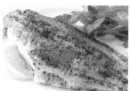

Coat both sides of fish filet with olive oil. For seasoning mixture combine the garlic powder, onion powder, cayenne pepper, paprika, salt, black pepper, thyme and cumin. Coat both sides of fish with the seasoning mixture.

Heat a heavy skillet (cast iron works good) over high heat. Once skillet is very hot, place fish in skillet. (Be sure to have the stove fan on, as I have personally set off my smoke alarm when preparing this dish). Cook 1 side 1 to 1 ½ minutes, then turn and cook other side 1 to 2 minutes or until done. Avoid overcooking which will dry the fish out. Fish continues to cook for several minutes after taken off the heat so I like to remove fish from the heat source when it is just a little underdone.

Serve immediately with lemon wedges.

Nutritional analysis per serving: 175 calories, 17 g. protein, 0 g. fiber, 11 g. fat, 9 mg. calcium, 402 mg. sodium.

Sautéed Yellow and Zucchini Squash Recipe:
For each serving:
1 tsp. olive oil
½ cup yellow squash, sliced or cut in matchsticks
½ cup zucchini squash, sliced or cut in matchsticks
1 clove garlic, chopped
1/8 tsp. sea salt
Black Pepper, to taste

Heat olive oil in skillet over medium heat. Add yellow squash and zucchini and cook 2 to 3 minutes. Add garlic and continue cooking just until squash is tender. Add salt and pepper and serve.

Nutritional Analysis per serving: 58 calories, 1 g. protein, 1 g. fiber, 5 g. fat, 18 mg. calcium, 296 mg. sodium.

Arugula Apricot Salad Recipe: May substitute other greens if you prefer milder greens.

Per person mix:
2 cups Arugula
4 Apricot halves
1/4 cup Radicchio, shredded
2 Tbsp. Balsamic Vinaigrette

To make Balsamic Vinaigrette put the following ingredients in a jar and shake until well blended:

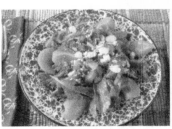

3 Tbsp. Balsamic vinegar
3 Tbsp. honey
1 Tbsp. plain, nonfat Greek yogurt
1 tsp. Dijon mustard
¼ cup olive or walnut oil

Top each salad with:
1 Tbsp. Gorgonzola Cheese
1 Tbsp. sliced almonds
If you can afford the extra calories add some avocado chunks

Nutritional analysis per serving not including avocado: 224 calories, 6 g. protein, 1 g. fiber, 14 g. fat, 142 mg. calcium, 155 mg. sodium.

Day 17 Menu

<u>Breakfast</u>
Almond Toast
2/3 Strawberry Smoothie
Beverage of Choice

<u>Lunch</u>
Shrimp Sweet Potato Cocktail
1/3 Strawberry Smoothie
Beverage of Choice

<u>Dinner</u>
Navy Bean Butternut Squash Soup
Spinach Pear Salad with Balsamic Vinaigrette
Beverage of Choice

If restricting sodium to 1500 mg/day: may add scant 1/8 tsp. salt to food or in cooking beyond what is already in the recipes.
2300 mg/day: may add an additional generous 3/8 tsp. salt to food or in cooking.

If not restricting calories to 1600/day:
Breakfast: May have 2nd almond toast.
Lunch: May have extra Shrimp cocktail and a serving whole grain bread.
Dinner: May have extra soup, salad and a serving of whole grain bread.

Recipes
Breakfast: Almond Toast, 2/3 Strawberry Smoothie.

Per person:
Spread 2 Tbsp. almond butter on 1 slice toasted whole grain bread.

Nutritional Analysis for 1 Almond Toast: 250 calories, 11 g. protein, 6 g. fiber, 17 g. fat, 110 mg. calcium, 112 mg. sodium.

Strawberry Smoothie Recipe: Drink 2/3's with Breakfast, and 1/3 with Lunch.

Per person blend all of the following ingredients in a high-speed blender until smooth:
3/4 cup of unsweetened Almond Milk (Calcium calculation based on
   using almond milk containing 300 mg calcium per 8 ounces or
   30% of the calcium RDA. If using a product higher than 300 mg.
   then use only amount of Almond Milk required for 300   mg.
   calcium and use water for the rest of the liquid).
½ cup plain nonfat Greek Yogurt (containing 300 mg calcium per 1
   cup serving. Nutrition label will say 30% of the RDA for calcium)
1 cup raw kale
1 cup raw spinach
1/2 cup frozen or fresh strawberries (may substitute another fruit for
   strawberries)
1 medium banana
1 Tbsp. flaxseed (optional, just adds 37 calories and has lots of
   health benefits)

Add additional water or ice cubes if a different consistency is desired. If you have parsley or other greens that you need to use before they go bad then add them to your smoothie – don't let them go to waste. If not limiting calories to 1600 per day may add additional fruits and vegetables.

Nutritional analysis per Smoothie: 266 calories, 18 g. protein, 7 g. fiber, 4 g. fat, 523 mg. calcium, 234 mg. sodium.

Lunch: Shrimp Sweet Potato Cocktail, 1/3 Strawberry Smoothie.

Shrimp Sweet Potato Cocktail Recipe: Makes 2 servings.
Preheat oven to 425° F.

1 sweet potato, cut into bite size pieces
1 cup pineapple chunks, fresh or canned in juice, drained
½ cup cherry tomatoes
1 tsp. olive oil
1 Tbsp. Balsamic vinegar (pineapple or regular)
1/8 tsp. cayenne pepper
6 ounces cooked shrimp
2 Tbsp. cilantro, chopped
2 Tbsp. red onion, chopped
1 jalapeno pepper, finely chopped
2 lime wedges
Avocado chunks, if not limiting calories to 1600/day

Mix sweet potato, pineapple and tomatoes with olive oil until well coated (works best to mix with hands). Add balsamic vinegar and cayenne pepper to mixture. Evenly distribute sweet potato, pineapple and tomato mixture on a parchment lined baking sheet. Roast at 425° F. for 20 to 25 minutes or until tomatoes pop or split and sweet potatoes are done.

Allow vegetable mixture to cool slightly then add shrimp, cilantro, red onion and jalapeno. Serve with lime wedges. If desired, add avocado chunks if not limiting calories to 1600/day.

Nutrient analysis per serving: 300 calories, 25 g. protein, 4 g. fiber, 4.5 g. fat, 109 mg. calcium and 546 mg. sodium.

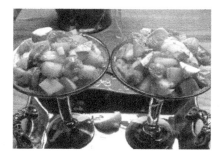

Dinner: Navy Bean Butternut Squash Soup, Spinach Pear Salad with Balsamic Vinaigrette.

Navy Bean Butternut Squash Soup Recipe: Makes 8 cups total, 4 servings of 2 cups each – make enough for Dinner and Lunch tomorrow.

1 medium onion, chopped
4 cloves garlic, minced
1 Tbsp. olive oil
2 14 ½ ounce cans or bottles no salt added diced tomatoes
2 cups water
1 12 ounce can beer (can use non-alcoholic beer)
1 tsp. ground cumin seed
1 Tbsp. fresh oregano, chopped or 1 tsp. dried oregano leaves
1 Tbsp. fresh thyme, chopped or 1 tsp. dried thyme
1/8 tsp. cayenne pepper, or to taste (I prefer to use ¼ tsp.)
¼ tsp. sea salt
2 15 oz. cans No salt added Navy Beans or 3 ½ cups cooked navy beans. I like Eden No Salt Added canned beans with BPA free lining or try Whole Foods 365 Organic No salt added beans that are packed in cartons. If you have time cook your own from dried beans.
3 cups butternut squash, coarsely chopped (may use frozen or fresh)
½ cup plain, nonfat Greek yogurt
2 Tbsp. lime juice
1 tsp. toasted cumin seed
4 lime wedges, optional

In a 4 quart pot heat olive oil over medium heat. Add onion and garlic and cook until tender. Mix in undrained canned tomatoes, water, beer, ground cumin seed, oregano, thyme, cayenne pepper and salt. Add undrained navy beans. Bring to boil, reduce heat. Add squash. Simmer, for 1 hour or until squash is tender. Stir frequently.

In batches transfer soup to blender and blend until smooth. CAUTION: Blending hot liquids will cause the lid of the blender to explode off. To avoid burns and a mess only fill the blender half full (blend in batches) and vent the lid. Many blenders have a lid with a center piece that comes out. Remove the center piece. Cover lid with kitchen towel to avoid sprays but still allow steam to escape. Thin with additional water if too thick. If you prefer a chunky soup then it is not necessary to blend the soup.

In small bowl mix yogurt and lime juice. Serve soup in bowls with 1/4th of yogurt mixture on top of each serving. Garnish top of yogurt with ¼ tsp. per serving cumin seed. If desired, can serve with lime wedges.

Nutritional analysis per serving: 411 calories, 19 g. protein, 4 g. fat, 19 g. fiber, 292 mg. calcium, 224 mg. sodium.

Spinach Pear Salad Recipe:

Per person mix:
2 cups Spinach
1 pear, cut into bite size pieces
¼ cup jicama, cut into bite size pieces
½ cup snow peas
2 Tbsp. Balsamic Vinaigrette

To make Balsamic Vinaigrette put the following ingredients in a jar and shake until well blended:
3 Tbsp. Balsamic vinegar
3 Tbsp. honey
1 Tbsp. plain, nonfat Greek yogurt
1 tsp. Dijon mustard
¼ cup olive or walnut oil

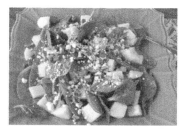

Top each salad with:
2 Tbsp. Goat Cheese
2 Tbsp. chopped pecans

Nutritional analysis per serving: 377 calories, 12 g. protein, 9 g. fiber, 24 g. fat, 177 mg. calcium, 149 mg. sodium.

Day 18 Menu

<u>Breakfast</u>
2 Apricot Quinoa Muffins
1 Egg cooked any way
½ Mango Smoothie
Beverage of Choice

<u>Lunch</u>
Navy Bean Butternut Squash Soup
½ cup Grapes or fruit of choice
½ Mango Smoothie
Beverage of Choice

<u>Dinner</u>
Roasted Chicken
Spaghetti Squash with Chutney
Swiss Chard
Strawberry "it's not really ice cream"
Beverage of Choice

If restricting sodium to 1500 mg/day: Do not add salt to food or in cooking beyond what is already in the recipes.
2300 mg/day: May add a scant additional 3/8 tsp. salt to food or in cooking.

If not restricting calories to 1600/day:
Breakfast: May have third muffin and second egg.
Lunch: May have extra soup and a serving of whole grain bread.
Dinner: May have 2 extra ounces chicken, a serving of whole grain bread and extra Strawberry "it's not really ice cream".

Recipes:
Breakfast: 2 Apricot Quinoa Muffins (leftover from Day 14), 1 Egg cooked any way, ½ Mango Smoothie.

Mango Smoothie Recipe: Drink ½ at Breakfast and ½ at Lunch.

Per person blend all of the following ingredients in a high-speed blender until smooth:
¼ cup of unsweetened Almond Milk (Calcium calculation based on using almond milk containing 300 mg calcium per 8 ounces or 30% of the calcium RDA. If using a product higher than 300 mg. then use only amount of Almond Milk required for 300 mg. calcium and use water for the rest of the liquid).
¾ cup plain nonfat Greek Yogurt (containing 300 mg calcium per 1 cup serving. Nutrition label will say 30% of the RDA for calcium)
1 cup raw kale
1 cup raw spinach
1/2 cup frozen or fresh mango (may substitute another fruit for mango)
1 medium banana
1 Tbsp. flaxseed (optional, just adds 37 calories and has lots of health benefits)

Add additional water or ice cubes if a different consistency is desired. If you have parsley or other greens that you need to use before they go bad then add them to your smoothie – don't let them go to waste. If not limiting calories to 1600 per day may add additional fruits and vegetables as desired.

Nutritional analysis per Smoothie without flaxseed: 306 calories, 23 g. protein, 7 g. fiber, 2 g. fat, 444 mg. calcium, 168 mg. sodium.

Lunch: Navy Bean Butternut Squash Soup (leftover from yesterday), ½ cup Grapes or fruit of choice, ½ Mango Smoothie.

Dinner: Roasted Chicken, Spaghetti Squash with Chutney, Swiss Chard, Strawberry "it's not really ice cream".

You can purchase already prepared Roasted or Rotisserie Chicken but try to purchase one that has not had a lot of salt and butter added to it.

Roast Chicken Recipe:

3 ½ to 4 pound chicken, preferably Organic free range
1 tsp. sea salt
¼ tsp. black pepper, ground
8 cloves garlic, 4 thinly sliced and 4 whole
5 sprigs fresh rosemary or 1 Tbsp. dried, and extra for cavity, if
    desired
1 organic lemon cut in fourths
olive oil

Season the chicken as soon as possible before cooking. You can season it the day before cooking or if you purchase the chicken the day of roasting season it as soon as you bring it home. To season remove the giblets from the cavity of the chicken. Mix salt and pepper and sprinkle all over chicken both inside and outside. Push garlic slices and rosemary under skin of chicken over breast and thighs. Put lemon and whole garlic in cavity of chicken. If desired add some extra rosemary sprigs to cavity of chicken. Tuck in wings.

When ready to roast preheat oven to 400° F. Use olive oil to lightly oil roasting pan that is about the same size as the chicken. Place chicken in pan breast side up and roast for 20 minutes. Turn chicken breast side down and roast for another 20 minutes. Turn chicken breast side up again and roast until done, about another 20 minutes. To test for doneness and to be sure the meat is no longer red cut into the bird near the joint between the drumstick and thigh. Do not overcook which dries chicken out.

Let chicken rest for 10 minutes before serving.

Nutritional Analysis per 3 ounce serving – no skin: 147 calories, 22 g. protein, 6 g. fat, 16 mg. calcium, 355 mg. sodium.

Spaghetti Squash with Chutney Recipe:
Serving size is 1 cup of squash.

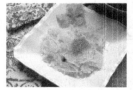

Preheat oven to 400° F.

Cut squash in half. Remove seeds. Place cut side down in a baking dish lightly oiled with olive oil. If not limiting calories to

1600/day may lightly brush squash with additional olive oil. Bake at 400° until tender when pierced with a fork, about 30 to 40 minutes. Remove from oven. Pull a fork lengthwise through the flesh to pull off spaghetti like long strands. Mix 1 tsp. butter and 1 Tbsp. chutney into each cup of squash. Serve immediately.

Nutritional analysis per serving: 102 calories, 1 g. protein, 2 g. fiber, 4 g. fat, 40 mg. calcium, 103 mg. sodium.

Swiss Chard Recipe:

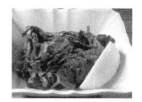

Per person:
In skillet over medium heat sauté 3 cups Swiss chard in 1 tsp. olive oil until tender. Add black pepper to taste. May also add fresh lemon juice if desired.

Nutritional analysis per serving: 60 calories, 2 g. protein, 2 g. fiber, 5 g. fat, 55 mg. calcium, 230 mg. sodium.

Strawberry "Not Really Ice Cream":

For each serving combine 1 cup slightly thawed frozen strawberries, ¼ cup plain, nonfat Greek yogurt and 2 tsp. maple syrup in a food processor. Blend until smooth. Serve immediately or if you want it more frozen put in freezer until desired consistency.

Nutrient analysis: 119 calories, 6 g. protein, 3 g. fiber, .2 g. fat, 108 mg. calcium, 28 mg sodium.

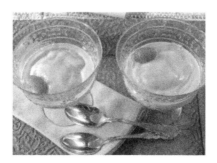

Day 19 Menu

Breakfast
Ricotta English Muffin with Strawberries
1 Egg cooked any way
Beverage of Choice

Lunch
Sweet Potato Black Bean Salad
Blueberry Smoothie
Beverage of Choice

Dinner
Fish Tacos
Fruit Salad
Beverage of Choice

If restricting sodium to 1500 mg/day: May add 1/16th tsp. salt to food or in cooking beyond what is already in the recipes.
2300 mg/day: May add an additional generous 3/8 tsp. salt to food or in cooking.

If not restricting calories to 1600/day:
Lunch: May have extra salad and a serving whole grain bread.
Dinner: May have avocado or guacamole.

Recipes
Breakfast: Ricotta English Muffin with Strawberries, 1 egg cooked any way.

English Muffin with Ricotta Cheese and Sliced Strawberries Recipe:

For each serving:
1 Whole grain English muffin
½ cup ricotta cheese
1 tsp. honey
4 medium strawberries, sliced

Split English muffin in half and toast if desired. Mix ricotta cheese with honey and spread evenly over 2 English muffin halves. Layer strawberries on top of cheese mixture.

Nutritional analysis per serving: 342 calories, 20 g. protein, 5 g. fiber, 11 g. fat, 520 mg. calcium, 396 mg. sodium.

Lunch: Sweet Potato Black Bean Salad, Blueberry Smoothie.

Sweet Potato Black Bean Salad Recipe: Makes 4 servings – half recipe for 2.

Preheat oven to 425°F.

1 sweet potato, cut into bite size slices (If you are halving the recipe to make 2 servings instead of 4 you can use the whole sweet potato)
1 tsp. olive oil
1 tsp. allspice
¼ tsp. cumin, ground
1/8 tsp. cayenne pepper
1 can 15 ounce can low sodium black beans, well drained (or 1 ¾ cup cooked)
½ tsp. Mexican oregano
¼ tsp. sea salt
2 Tbsp. chopped cilantro, chopped
1 ½ cups grated carrot
1 orange divided into bite size sections

1 stalk celery, chopped
¼ cup pumpkin seeds
2 Avocados
¼ cup Feta cheese

Dressing:
1 ½ tsp. Dijon mustard
2 Tbsp. lime juice
1 Tbsp. maple syrup
2 Tbsp. olive oil

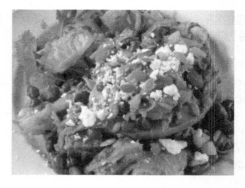

Mix sweet potato with 1 tsp. olive oil. Mix sweet potato with allspice, cumin and cayenne pepper. Distribute evenly on a parchment lined baking pan. Roast at 425° for 20 to 30 minutes or until tender. Set aside to cool.

In large bowl, mix black beans, oregano, salt, cilantro, carrot, orange, celery and pumpkin seeds.

To make dressing mix Dijon mustard, lime juice, maple syrup and olive oil in a jar. Shake until well blended.

Serve salad in avocado half. (It won't all fit in the avocado half so just serve the rest on the plate with the avocado. Top with feta cheese.

Nutritional Analysis per serving: 492 calories, 13 g. protein, 16 g. fiber, 30 g. fat, 168 mg. calcium, 373 mg. sodium.

Blueberry Smoothie Recipe: Drink with Lunch.

Per person blend all of the following ingredients in a high-speed blender until smooth:
¼ cup of unsweetened Almond Milk (Calcium calculation based on
    using almond milk containing 300 mg calcium per 8 ounces or
    30% of the calcium RDA. If using a product higher than 300
    mg.then use only amount of Almond Milk required for 300 mg.
    calcium and use water for the rest of the liquid).
½ cup plain nonfat Greek Yogurt (containing 300 mg calcium per 1
    cup serving. Nutrition label will say 30% of the RDA for calcium)
½ cup raw kale

½ cup frozen or fresh blueberries (may substitute another fruit for blueberries)
1 medium banana
1 Tbsp. flaxseed (optional, just adds 37 calories and has lots of health benefits)

Add additional water or ice cubes if a different consistency is desired. If you have parsley or other greens that you need to use before they go bad then add them to your smoothie – don't let them go to waste. If not limiting calories to 1600 per day may add additional fruits and vegetables as desired.

Nutritional analysis per Smoothie: 236 calories, 15 g. protein, 6 g. fiber, 2 g. fat, 287 mg. calcium, 107 mg. sodium.

Dinner: Fish Tacos, Fruit Salad.

Fish Tacos Recipe: Serves 4 – serving is 2 tacos.
For fish, preferably purchase sustainable fish such as Arctic Char (farmed), Tilapia (Equador & US), Catfish (US) or Pacific Halibut (US). Go to www.seafoodwatch.org for sustainable fish purchasing guidelines. You can also look for fish with the Marine Stewardship Council Blue eco-label in your grocery store.

Sauce:
1 cup plain nonfat Greek yogurt
1/8 tsp. cayenne pepper
1 tsp. fresh lime juice
1/8 tsp. cumin seed, ground
2 Tbsp. cilantro, chopped
¼ tsp. sea salt
2 tsp. honey
1/8 tsp. chili powder, more if you like a spicier, hotter sauce

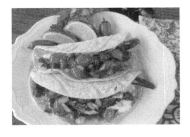

For sauce: In small bowl mix yogurt, cayenne pepper, lime juice, cumin, cilantro, salt, honey and chili powder.

Pico de Gallo:
2 Tbsp. cilantro, chopped
2 Tbsp. chopped onion
1 jalapeno, chopped finely

½ cup chopped tomato
1 clove garlic, minced

For pico de gallo: In small bowl mix cilantro, onion, jalapeno, tomato and garlic.

Fish:
1 pound fish, cut in to ½" pieces
¼ cup cilantro, chopped
¼ tsp. sea salt
1/4 tsp. cumin seed, ground
1/4 tsp. chili powder
2 tsp. olive oil

In a medium bowl mix fish, cilantro, salt, cumin seed and chili powder together.   Heat olive oil over medium heat in large skillet. Cook fish until done, about 3 to 5 minutes.

2 cups shredded cabbage
8 corn tortillas – warmed
4 lime wedges

Serve fish in tortillas with shredded cabbage, sauce and pico de gallo with lime wedges on the side.

Nutritional Analysis for 2 Fish Tacos: 290 calories, 32 g. protein, 4 g. fiber, 6 g. fat, 152 mg. calcium, 411 mg. sodium.

Fruit Salad Recipe:

Per Person:
Mix the following fruits together as a salad – may substitute other in season fruits. Garnish with fresh mint if desired:

1 cup watermelon – cut in bite size chunks
¼ cup fresh blueberries
½ cup cantaloupe – cut in bite size chunks
½ cup blackberries

Nutritional analysis per serving: 128 calories, 3 g. protein, 7 g. fiber, 0 g. fat, 42 mg. calcium, 16 mg. sodium.

Day 20 Menu

Breakfast
Pumpkin Waffles with Strawberries
1/3 Peach Smoothie
Beverage of Choice

Lunch
Hummus with Crackers and Raw Vegetables
2/3 Peach Smoothie
Grapefruit half or Fruit of choice
Beverage of Choice

Dinner
Bison Meatloaf
Baked Sweet Potato
Roasted Green Beans
Orange or Fruit of choice
Beverage of Choice

If restricting sodium to 1500 mg/day: Do not add salt to food or in cooking beyond what is already in the recipes.
2300 mg./day: May add an additional generous ¼ tsp. salt to food or in cooking.

If not restricting calories to 1600/day:
Breakfast: May have extra waffles.
Lunch: May have extra hummus and vegetables.
Dinner: May have extra serving meatloaf, and a serving of whole grain bread.

Recipes:
Breakfast: Pumpkin Waffles with Strawberries, 1/3 Peach Smoothie.

Pumpkin Waffles with Strawberries Recipe: Makes 10 waffles (may vary according to waffle iron) – serving size is 1 waffle.

Preheat waffle iron.

Topping **per person**:
½ cup fat free, plain Greek Yogurt
2 Tbsp. 100% maple syrup
1/8 tsp. allspice
1/8 tsp. cinnamon
1/8 tsp. cloves
Waffles:
1 cup whole wheat flour
¾ cup all purpose, unbleached flour
1 Tbsp. ground flax seed
¼ tsp. allspice, ground
½ tsp. cinnamon, ground
¼ tsp. cloves, ground
1/8 tsp. nutmeg, ground
¼ tsp. ginger, ground
2 tsp. baking powder
½ tsp. salt
2 eggs
1 cup canned pumpkin*
1 ½ cups skim milk
¼ cup canola oil (preferably organic)
1 Tbsp. honey or maple syrup
1 tsp. vanilla extract

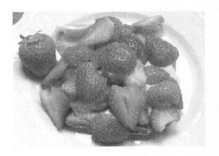

1 cup sliced strawberries **per person**

To make topping mix yogurt, maple syrup, allspice, cinnamon and cloves. Use less of the spices if you prefer a less spicy topping. Set aside until ready to top and serve waffles.

In medium bowl, mix flours, flax seed, allspice, cinnamon, cloves, nutmeg, ginger, baking powder and salt.

In medium bowl, mix eggs, pumpkin, milk, canola oil, honey and vanilla until well blended. Fold the flour mixture into the pumpkin mixture.

Cook waffles in waffle iron until brown and crisp. Top with yogurt mixture and sliced strawberries.

Nutritional analysis per serving: 394 calories, 19 g. protein, 6 g. fiber, 7 grams fat, 324 mg. calcium, 300 mg. sodium

* Use leftover pumpkin in Smoothies. To make a Pumpkin Smoothie, mix leftover pumpkin with Greek yogurt, ground cinnamon, cloves and ginger and add a couple of dates with the seeds removed. I include some spinach to make it even more nutritious and a little squeeze of lemon juice as well. If you want additional sweetness add a banana.

Peach Smoothie Recipe: Drink 1/3 with Breakfast and 2/3's with Lunch.

Per person blend all of the following ingredients in a high-speed blender until smooth:
¾ cup of unsweetened Almond Milk (Calcium calculation based on using almond milk containing 300 mg calcium per 8 ounces or 30% of the calcium RDA. If using a product higher than 300 mg. then use only amount of Almond Milk required for 300 mg. calcium and use water for the rest of the liquid).
¾ cup plain nonfat Greek Yogurt (containing 300 mg calcium per 1 cup serving. Nutrition label will say 30% of the RDA for calcium)
1 cup raw kale
1/2 cup frozen or fresh peach slices (may substitute another fruit for peach)
1 medium banana
1 Tbsp. flaxseed (optional, just adds 37 calories and has lots of health benefits)

Add additional water or ice cubes if a different consistency is desired. If you have parsley or other greens that you need to use before they go bad then add them to your smoothie – don't let them go to waste. If not restricting calories to 1600 per day you may add additional fruits and vegetables as desired.

Nutritional analysis for 1 Smoothie not including flaxseed: 314 calories, 23 g. protein, 7 g. fiber, 4 g. fat, 564 mg. calcium, 233 mg. sodium.

Lunch: Hummus with Crackers and Raw Vegetables, 2/3 Peach Smoothie, Grapefruit half or fruit of choice.

You can make your own homemade hummus or purchase it already made. Try a variety of brands to determine which one you like best.

For Lunch:
1/2 cup Hummus with as many raw vegetables as you like.
Try: Broccoli, Cauliflower, Carrot Sticks, Cucumbers, Red or Yellow Pepper slices, Celery
6 whole grain crackers (I like Flackers – crackers made from flax seeds or try Multigrain Wasa Flatbreads) or a slice of whole grain bread.

Dinner: Bison Meatloaf, Baked Sweet Potato, Roasted Green Beans, Orange or fruit of choice.

Bison Meatloaf Recipe: Serves 8.
Preheat oven to 400° F.

2 lbs. ground Bison meat (may substitute 95% lean, 5% fat ground
    beef but if you haven't tried Bison you should. Many grocery
    stores now carry Bison.)
2 green onions, chopped
1 tsp. dried oregano
½ tsp. sea salt
1 tsp. black pepper
1 Tbsp. Garlic powder
1 tsp. paprika (regular or smoked)
¼ cup parsley, chopped
¼ cup fresh basil, chopped or 1 Tbsp. dried basil
2 cups tomato sauce, divided into ½ cup and 1 ½ cups
2 eggs
1 cup rolled oats (not instant)
¼ cup water

Mix meat, onions, oregano, salt, pepper, garlic powder, paprika, parsley and basil. Add eggs and ½ cup tomato sauce. Add rolled oats and mix until well blended.

Form in to loaf in oil sprayed baking pan and top with remaining 1 ½ cup tomato sauce. Add ¼ cup water to pan and bake uncovered at 400° for 45 minutes or until done. Best to let it sit 10 minutes before slicing.

Nutritional analysis per serving: 245 calories, 27 g. protein, 3 g. fiber, 10 g. fat, 46 mg. calcium, 568 mg. sodium.

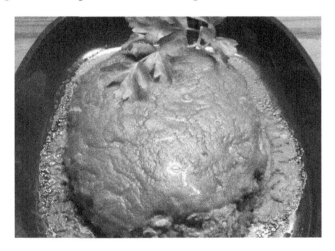

Baked Sweet Potato Recipe:

1 sweet potato per person. Scrub well and bake at 425° F. for 1 hour or until done. Pierce with fork after sweet potato has been in the oven for 30 minutes. If you have more than 1 tsp. of butter on the potato you will exceed 1600 calories for the day. I don't advocate the use of butter on a regular basis but there are certain foods that warrant butter and in my opinion a baked sweet potato is one of them.

Nutritional analysis for 1 medium baked Sweet Potato with 1 tsp. salted butter: 137 calories, 2 g. protein, 5 g. fiber, 4 g. fat, 43 mg. calcium, 75 mg. sodium.

Roasted Green Beans Recipe:
Preheat oven to 400°F.
For each serving:
1 cup green beans, stem ends cut off
1 tsp. olive oil
Black pepper to taste
1 tsp. fresh thyme, chopped
1 Tbsp. toasted sliced almonds, if not limiting calories to 1600
    calories/day

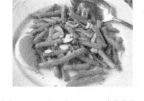

Place green beans in bowl. Add olive oil to coat green beans (if you use your hands it will coat more evenly). Add black pepper. Evenly distribute green beans in a single layer on a parchment lined baking pan. Bake at 400° F. for 8 to 10 minutes or until done, stirring once after 5 minutes. Sprinkle with thyme just before serving. If you can afford an additional 33 calories, sprinkle 1 Tbsp. almond slices on top as well.

Alternative Cooking method: If you have good quality green beans (fresh from Farmer's Market or your own garden) or haricots verts then you can simply boil them or sauté them until done and add seasonings. When standard grocery store green beans are all that is available to you then roasting is often a better preparation method.

Nutritional Analysis per serving not including almonds: 70 calories, 2 g. protein, 3 g. fiber, 5 g. fat, 38 mg. calcium, 6 mg. sodium.

Day 21 Menu

Breakfast
Sweet Potato Egg Scramble
1 slice Whole Grain Toast with jam
Beverage of Choice

Lunch
Salmon Salad in Avocado Half
Pineapple Smoothie
Beverage of Choice

Dinner
Carrot Farro Risotto
Kale with Raisins and Pine Nuts
Greek Yogurt with warm Berry Compote
Beverage of Choice

If restricting sodium to 1500 mg/day: Do not add salt to food or in cooking beyond what is already in the recipes.
2300 mg/day: May add an additional generous ¼ tsp. salt to food or in cooking.

If not restricting calories to 1600/day:
Breakfast: May have extra eggs, second slice of toast or whole grain biscuits instead of toast.
Lunch: May have extra salmon salad and a serving of whole grain bread.
Dinner: May have extra Risotto, a serving whole grain bread and extra Yogurt with Berry Compote.

Recipes:
Breakfast: Sweet Potato Egg Scramble, 1 slice whole grain toast with jam.

Sweet Potato Egg Scramble Recipe: Serves 2

4 large eggs (may substitute 8 egg
    whites or 2 eggs plus 4 egg whites)
¼ tsp. ground cumin
¼ tsp. smoked paprika
1/8 tsp. sea salt
1/8 tsp. cayenne pepper (optional)
1 tsp. olive oil
1 medium sweet potato, peeled and
    sliced into bite size pieces
8 cups fresh spinach

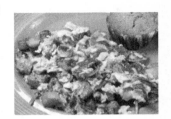

In small bowl whisk together eggs, cumin, paprika, salt and cayenne pepper. Set aside.

In medium skillet heat olive oil over medium heat. Add sweet potato. Cook, stirring frequently, until done, about 10 to 12 minutes. Add spinach, cook until just wilted, about 1 to 2 minutes. Reduce heat to low. Add egg mixture. Cook, stirring frequently, until eggs are just done, about 2 to 3 minutes. Serve immediately.

To speed up preparation you can roast the sweet potato in 1 tsp. olive oil ahead of time at 425° F. for 20 to 25 minutes. When ready to prepare dish heat sweet potato in skillet until warm. Then add spinach and cook until spinach is just wilted. Then add eggs cooking until done.

Nutritional analysis per serving: 246 calories, 17 g. protein, 5 g. fiber, 12 g. fat, 194 mg. calcium, 418 mg. sodium.
If you roast the sweet potato and use an extra tsp. of olive oil the calories will increase to 266 and fat will increase to 15 g.

Lunch: Salmon Salad in Avocado half, Pineapple Smoothie.

Salmon Salad in Avocado Half Recipe: Makes 2 servings.

1 6-ounce can wild salmon
1 Tbsp. basil pesto – if not available then mix 2 Tbsp. chopped basil
    with a little olive oil
1 Tbsp. canola or olive oil mayonnaise
1/8 tsp. garlic powder
1 tsp. minced red onion
1 Tbsp. minced celery
1 Tbsp. fresh squeezed lemon juice
1 tsp. white wine vinegar (may   substitute apple cider vinegar)
Black pepper to taste
1 jalapeno, finely chopped (optional – may leave out or use less)
1 ripe avocado, halved with pit removed

In a small bowl, mix all ingredients except the avocado with a fork.
Leave the jalapeno out if you don't want the addition of hot pepper.
Spoon salmon salad into avocado halves.

Nutritional analysis per serving: 371 calories, 24 g. protein, 7 g.
fiber, 28 g. fat, 85 mg. calcium, 427 mg sodium.

Pineapple Smoothie Recipe: Drink with Lunch.

Per person blend all of the following ingredients in a high-speed
blender until smooth:
1 cup of unsweetened Almond Milk (Calcium calculation based on
    using almond milk containing 300 mg calcium per 8 ounces or
    30% of the calcium RDA. If using a product higher than 300 mg.
    then use only amount of Almond Milk required for 300 mg.
    calcium and use water for the rest of the liquid).
1 cup raw kale
½ cup frozen, canned or fresh pineapple (may substitute another
    fruit for pineapple)
1 medium banana
1 Tbsp. flaxseed (optional, just adds 37 calories and has lots of
    health benefits)

Add additional water or ice cubes if a different consistency is desired. If you have parsley or other greens that you need to use before they go bad then add them to your smoothie – don't let them go to waste. If not restricting calories to 1600 per day you may add additional fruits and vegetables as desired.

Nutritional analysis per serving not including flaxseed: 215 calories, 6 g. protein, 5 g. fiber, 4 g. fat, 417 mg. calcium, 208 mg. sodium.

Dinner: Carrot Farro Risotto, Kale with Raisins and Pine Nuts, Greek Yogurt with warm Berry Compote.

Carrot Farro Risotto Recipe: Makes 4 servings.
Preheat oven to 400° F.

10 ounces carrots, washed and sliced into bite size pieces
1 tsp. plus 1 Tbsp. olive oil, divided
½ tsp. ground coriander, divided
½ tsp. ground cumin, divided
½ cup water
1 cup Farro
2 cloves garlic, finely chopped
½ cup white wine
2 ½ cups low sodium vegetable broth
¼ tsp. sea salt
2 Tbsp. pistachios (may substitute almonds, walnuts, pine nuts or
    pecans)
2 Tbsp. flat leaf parsley or cilantro

Coat carrots with 1 tsp. olive oil, ¼ tsp. coriander and ¼ tsp. cumin. It works best to use your hands. Evenly distribute carrots on parchment lined baking sheet and cook for 20 to 25 minutes at 400° F. or until tender. Stir half way through cooking time. Remove from oven when done. Allow carrots to cool a few minutes. Set aside ½ cup of sliced carrots. In a blender or food processor puree remaining carrots with water, ¼ tsp. coriander and ¼ tsp. cumin until smooth. Add additional water as needed to get a smooth puree.

In medium saucepan warm vegetable broth over low heat. Keep warm.

In a separate medium saucepan, heat 1 Tbsp. olive oil over low heat. Sauté farro and garlic in olive oil for 1 minute, stirring constantly. Add white wine and stir until wine is absorbed. Add ½ cup of warm vegetable broth and stir frequently until broth is absorbed. Continue adding ½ cup of warm vegetable broth and stirring frequently until broth has absorbed. It should be done in 30 to 40 minutes. You can add additional water or broth if it needs more liquid.

Add pureed carrots, sliced carrots, salt, pistachios and parsley (or cilantro) to farro. Cook until warm, stirring constantly.

Alternative Easy version:
Roast carrots with seasonings. Make farro according to package directions, substituting broth and wine for liquid. Add seasonings. Mix roasted carrots, pistachios, parsley and farro together.

Nutritional analysis per serving: 299 calories, 9 g. protein, 8 g. fiber, 8 g. fat, 62 mg. calcium, 286 mg. sodium.

Kale with Raisins and Pine Nuts Recipe:

Per person:
2 cups kale, washed and torn into bite size pieces with ribs removed
1 tsp. olive oil
2 Tbsp. raisins
1 Tbsp. pine nuts

Heat olive oil in skillet over medium heat. Add kale and cook, stirring frequently, until just wilted. Add raisins and pine nuts. Serve immediately.

Nutritional analysis per serving: 216 calories, 8 g. protein, 4 g. fiber, 11 g. fat, 210 mg. calcium, 53 mg. sodium.

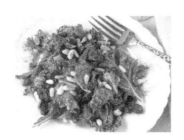

Greek Yogurt with Warm Berry Compote Recipe:

Per Person:
½ cup Greek yogurt
2 tsp. honey – divided
1 cup mixed berries – raspberries, blueberries, strawberries,
  blackberries
¼ cup orange juice (nutritional analysis includes calcium added
  orange juice)
1 tsp. balsamic vinegar or favorite liqueur, like Grand Marnier or
  Crème de Cassis (optional)

Mix Greek yogurt with 1 tsp. honey. Put in freezer while preparing
compote.

In saucepan, mix berries with 1 tsp. honey and orange juice. Over
medium heat, bring to a boil, reduce heat to low and cook, stirring
frequently, until reduced and thickened, about 10 minutes. Add
balsamic vinegar or liqueur, if desired. Remove yogurt from freezer
and transfer to serving container. Pour fruit over yogurt. Eat
immediately.

Nutritional analysis per serving: 203 calories, 13 g. protein, 6 g.
fiber, .8 g. fat, 256 mg. calcium, 53 mg sodium.

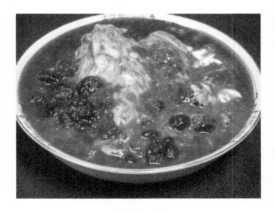

Day 22 Menu

Breakfast
Granola with Strawberries
Beverage of Choice

Lunch
Pear Quinoa Salad
½ Mango Smoothie
Beverage of Choice

Dinner
Vegetable Biryani
½ Mango Smoothie
Beverage of Choice

If restricting sodium to 1500 mg/day: May add scant 3/8 tsp. salt to food or in cooking beyond what is already in the recipes.
2300 mg/day: May add an additional generous 5/8 tsp. salt to food or in cooking.

If not restricting calories to 1600/day:
All meals: May have extra servings of everything plus a serving whole grain bread at both Lunch and Dinner.
Dinner: May add chutney to Vegetable Biryani.

Recipes:
Breakfast: Granola with Strawberries.

½ cup Granola with ¾ cup Non-fat Plain Greek Yogurt, ½ cup sliced strawberries and 1 tsp. honey or maple syrup if desired. May substitute another fruit for strawberries. You will need to make the Granola before the morning you plan to eat it. Store it for future use. Granola recipe is on Day 5.

Lunch: Pear Quinoa Salad, ½ Mango Smoothie.

Pear and Arugula Quinoa Salad Recipe: Serves 4 – make enough to have for Lunch twice this week.

1 cup quinoa, rinsed
2 ½ cups water
2 ripe pears, cut in to bite size pieces
4 cups arugula
2 Tbsp. Italian parsley, chopped
½ cup dried cherries, chopped
½ cup walnuts, chopped and toasted

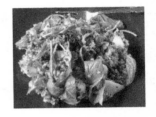

Dressing:
4 Tbsp. olive oil
3 Tbsp. balsamic vinegar
2 Tbsp. maple syrup

Rinse quinoa well. Bring water to a boil in a medium saucepan. Mix in quinoa and reduce heat to low. Cover and cook until done, about 15 to 20 minutes.

To make dressing mix olive oil, vinegar and maple syrup together.

In a large bowl, mix quinoa, pears, arugula, parsley, dried cherries and walnuts. Add dressing and mix lightly until all ingredients are coated with dressing.

Nutritional analysis per serving: 464 calories, 9 g. protein, 7 g. fiber, 26 g. fat, 82 mg. calcium, 13 mg. sodium.

Mango Smoothie Recipe: Drink ½ with Lunch and ½ with Dinner.

Per person blend all of the following ingredients in a high-speed blender until smooth:

½ cup of unsweetened Almond Milk (Calcium calculation based on using almond milk containing 300 mg calcium per 8 ounces or 30% of the calcium RDA. If using a product higher than 300 mg. then use only amount of Almond Milk required for 300 mg. calcium and use water for the rest of the liquid).

¾ cup plain nonfat Greek Yogurt (containing 300 mg calcium per 1 cup serving. Nutrition label will say 30% of the RDA for calcium)

2 cups raw kale

½ cup frozen or fresh mango (may substitute another fruit for mango)

1 medium banana

1 Tbsp. flaxseed (optional, just adds 37 calories and has lots of health benefits)

Add additional water or ice cubes if a different consistency is desired. If you have parsley or other greens that you need to use before they go bad then add them to your smoothie – don't let them go to waste. If not limiting calories to 1600 per day you may add additional fruits and vegetables as desired.

Nutritional analysis per serving without flaxseed: 342 calories, 25 g. protein, 8 g. fiber, 3 g. fat, 590 mg. calcium, 215 mg. sodium.

Dinner: Vegetable Biryani, ½ Mango Smoothie.

Vegetable Biryani with Barley Recipe: Makes 4 servings – make enough for lunch tomorrow.

For the Barley:
1 cup hulled barley, may use pearl if hulled not available
¼ tsp. salt
1/8 tsp. cayenne pepper
1 ½ tsp. turmeric
¾ tsp. ground cumin
¾ tsp. ground coriander
¾ tsp. ground cardamom
¾ tsp. ground cinnamon

2 Tbsp. sliced almonds
¼ cup raisins

For the topping:
1 cup Greek Yogurt
3 strands saffron (if saffron is not available then substitute ¼ tsp. turmeric)
¼ cup cilantro, chopped

For the Vegetables:
1 Tbsp. olive oil
1 medium yellow onion, diced
3 cloves garlic, minced
1 Tbsp. peeled minced ginger
¼ cup raisins
2 Tbsp. sliced almonds
1/8 tsp. cayenne pepper
1 ½ tsp. ground coriander
¾ tsp. ground cumin
½ tsp. ground cardamom
2 cups bite size broccoli florets
2 cups bite size cauliflower florets
2 medium carrots, sliced into bite size pieces
1 cup green beans, cut into bite size pieces
¼ tsp. salt
½ cup water

Chutney (optional and if not limiting calories to 1600/day)

In medium saucepan bring 4 cups water to a boil. Add barley and reduce heat to low. Cover and cook until done and water has all been absorbed, about 1 hour. Mix cayenne pepper, turmeric, cumin, coriander, cardamom, cinnamon, almonds and raisins in to barley.

Mix yogurt with saffron, or turmeric, and cilantro. Set aside.

Heat olive oil in large skillet (one that has a lid) over medium heat. Add the onion and cook until lightly browned, stirring frequently. Add the garlic and ginger and cook, stirring constantly, about 1 minute. Mix the raisins, almonds, cayenne pepper, coriander, cumin, and cardamom in and cook about 1 minute. Add the broccoli, cauliflower, carrots, green beans and salt to the skillet. Stir in water, cover and cook for 5 minutes. Uncover and stir and cook until vegetables are just done (not mushy) and water has evaporated.

Serve vegetables over rice. Top each serving with ¼ cup yogurt sauce and a spoonful of chutney if desired (chutney is optional).

Nutritional Analysis per serving not including chutney: 407 calories, 18 g. protein, 15 g. fiber, 8 g. fat, 210 mg. calcium and 385 mg. sodium.

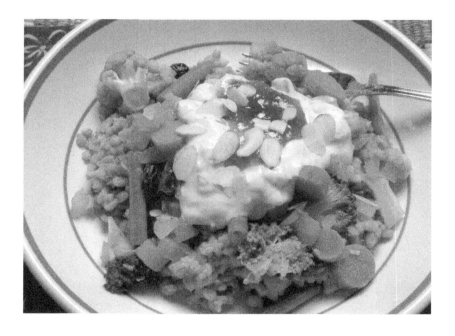

Day 23 Menu

Breakfast
Oatmeal with Pineapple and Walnuts
1/3 of Cherry Smoothie
Beverage of Choice

Lunch
Vegetable Biryani
2/3's of Cherry Smoothie
Beverage of Choice

Dinner
Grilled/Baked Salmon in Apricot Oregano Sauce
Roasted Broccoli
Spinach Cranberry Salad
Beverage of Choice

If restricting sodium to 1500 mg/day: May add scant ¼ tsp. salt to food or in cooking beyond what is already in the recipes.
2300 mg/day: May add generous ½ tsp. salt to food or in cooking.

If not restricting calories to 1600/day:
Breakfast: May have additional oatmeal and fruit.
Lunch: May have additional Vegetable Biryani with chutney and a serving whole grain bread.
Dinner: May have 2 extra ounces of salmon, a serving whole grain bread and avocado in the salad.

Recipes
Breakfast: Oatmeal with Pineapple and Walnuts, 1/3 Cherry Smoothie.

Oatmeal with Pineapple and Walnuts Recipe: Makes 1 serving.

¼ cup steel cut oats (may substitute rolled oats if you prefer)
1 cup unsweetened almond milk
¼ tsp. ground cinnamon, or to taste
1/8 tsp. ground ginger, or to taste
½ tsp. vanilla, or to taste
1 tsp. honey or maple syrup
1 Tbsp. flaxseed (optional, just adds 37 calories and has lots of
     health benefits)
½ cup chopped pineapple
1 Tbsp. walnuts, chopped

Prepare oatmeal according to package directions using almond milk instead of water. Mix in cinnamon, ginger, vanilla, honey (or maple syrup) and flaxseed. Once cooked to desired consistency add pineapple and walnuts and serve immediately. If not restricting calories to 1600 per day may have more pineapple and walnuts.

Nutritional analysis per serving not including flaxseed: 328 calories, 10 g. protein, 9 g. fiber, 8 g. fat, 341 mg. calcium, 182 mg. sodium

Cherry Smoothie Recipe: Drink 1/3 with Breakfast and 2/3's with Lunch.

Cherry Smoothie Recipe:
Per person blend all of the following ingredients in a high-speed blender until smooth:
1/3 cup unsweetened Almond Milk (Calcium calculation based on
     using almond milk containing 300 mg calcium per 8 ounces or
     30% of the calcium RDA. If using a product higher than 300 mg.
     then use only amount of Almond Milk required for 300 mg.
     calcium and use water for the rest of the liquid).
1 cup plain nonfat Greek Yogurt (containing 300 mg calcium per 1
     cup serving. Nutrition label will say 30% of the RDA for calcium)
½ cup frozen cherries
½ cup beets (fresh or frozen)

1 cup spinach
1 medium banana
1 Tbsp. ground flaxseed (optional, just adds 37 calories and has lots
   of health benefits)

Add additional water or ice cubes if a different consistency is desired.

Nutritional Analysis per Smoothie not including flaxseed: 320 calories, 27 g. protein, 7 g. fiber, 2 g. fat, 457 mg. calcium and 234 mg. sodium.

Lunch: Vegetable Biryani (leftover from dinner yesterday), 2/3's Cherry Smoothie.

Dinner: Grilled/Baked Salmon in Apricot Oregano Sauce, Roasted Broccoli, Spinach Cranberry Salad.

Salmon in Apricot Oregano Sauce Recipe: Makes 4 servings.

Preheat oven to 400° F. if not grilling salmon.

1 pound raw salmon, preferably wild. Go to www.seafoodwatch.org
   for sustainable fish purchasing guidelines.   You can also look for
   fish with the Marine Stewardship Council Blue eco-label in your
   grocery store.
½ cup white wine or water if not grilling
½ cup apricot preserves (preferably a 100% fruit version)
3 Tbsp. green onions, chopped
1 ½ tsp. fresh oregano or ½ tsp. dried oregano

Mix apricot preserves, green onions and oregano in small bowl. Spread on top of salmon.

Cook salmon on grill until just done.   Or put in baking dish, add white wine or water and bake uncovered at 400° for 12 to 15 minutes or until just done.   Avoid overcooking which will dry the salmon out.   Fish continues to cook for several minutes after taken off the heat so some cooks like to remove fish from the heat source when it is just a little underdone.

Nutritional analysis per serving: 264 calories, 25 g. protein, 7 g. fat, 54 mg. calcium, 69 mg. sodium.

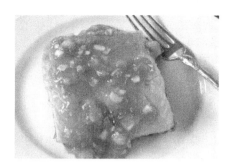

Roasted Broccoli Recipe:
Preheat oven to 400° F.

Per person:
1 cup broccoli, washed and cut into bite size florets
1 tsp. olive oil
Black pepper to taste or use red pepper flakes
1/8 tsp. garlic powder, if desired
Lemon juice/wedges, if desired or use red wine vinegar
Toasted almonds, if not restricting calories to 1600 per day

Place broccoli in bowl. Add olive oil to coat broccoli (if you use your hands it will coat more evenly). Add pepper, garlic and any other desired herbs or spices – oregano, thyme, caraway seeds, coriander or tarragon work well. Evenly distribute broccoli in a single layer on a parchment lined baking pan. Bake at 400° F. for 10 to 15 minutes or until done, stirring once after 5 minutes and again as needed. Squeeze fresh lemon juice over before serving.

Nutritional analysis per serving: 70 calories, 3 g. protein, 2 g. fiber, 5 g. fat, 43 mg. calcium, 30 mg. sodium.

If not restricting calories to 1600 per day sprinkle some toasted almonds on top of the Roasted Broccoli.

Spinach Cranberry Salad Recipe:

Per person mix:
2 cups spinach
½ apple, cut into bite size pieces
1 Tbsp. dried cranberries
1 Tbsp. chopped red onion
2 Tbsp. Maple Vinaigrette
Sunflower seeds if not limiting to 1600 calories/day

To make Maple Vinaigrette put the following ingredients in a jar and shake until well blended:

2 Tbsp. apple cider vinegar
2 Tbsp. maple syrup
1 Tbsp. Dijon mustard
2 Tbsp. olive oil

If not limiting calories to 1600/day top salad with some sunflower seeds.

Nutritional analysis per serving not including sunflower seeds: 187 calories, 2 g. protein, 3 g. fiber, 8 g. fat, 72 mg. calcium, 99 mg. sodium.

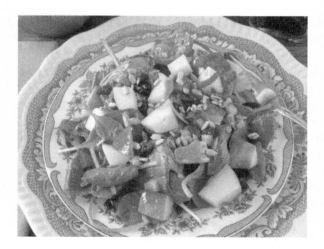

Day 24 Menu

Breakfast
Almond Toast
½ Raspberry Smoothie
Beverage of Choice

Lunch
Pear Quinoa Salad
½ Raspberry Smoothie
Beverage of Choice

Dinner
Filet Mignon
Roasted Brussels Sprouts with
Cranberries and Walnuts
Sautéed Swiss Chard
Orange or Fruit of Choice
Beverage of Choice

If restricting sodium to 1500 mg/day: May add 1/8 tsp. salt to food or in cooking beyond what is already in the recipes.
2300 mg/day: May add an additional 1/2 tsp. salt to food or in cooking.

If not restricting calories to 1600/day:
Breakfast: May have second Almond Toast.
Lunch: May have additional quinoa salad and a serving whole grain bread.
Dinner: May have an additional 2 ounces filet, a serving whole grain bread and may dip orange in melted dark chocolate or eat with a piece of chocolate.

Recipes
Breakfast: Almond Toast, ½ Raspberry Smoothie.

Per person:
Spread 2 Tbsp. almond butter on 1 slice toasted whole grain bread.

Nutritional Analysis for 1 Almond Toast: 250 calories, 11 g. protein, 6 g. fiber, 17 g. fat, 110 mg. calcium, 112 mg. sodium.

Raspberry Smoothie Recipe: Drink ½ with Breakfast and ½ with Lunch.

Per person blend all of the following ingredients in a high-speed blender until smooth:
1 cup of unsweetened Almond Milk (Calcium calculation based on
    using almond milk containing 300 mg calcium per 8 ounces
    or 30% of the calcium RDA. If using a product higher than 300
    mg. then use only amount of Almond Milk required for 300 mg.
    calcium and use water for the rest of the liquid).
1 cup plain nonfat Greek yogurt (containing 300 mg calcium per 1
    cup serving. Nutrition label will say 30% of the RDA for calcium)
1 cup raw kale
1 cup raw spinach
1 cup frozen or fresh raspberries (may substitute another fruit for
    raspberries)
1 medium banana
1 Tbsp. flaxseed (optional, just adds 37 calories and has lots of
    health benefits)

Add additional water or ice cubes if a different consistency is desired. If you have parsley or other greens that you need to use before they go bad then add them to your smoothie – don't let them go to waste. If not limiting calories to 1600 per day may add additional fruits and vegetables as desired.

Nutritional analysis per Smoothie: 445 calories, 32 g. protein, 22 g. fiber, 6 g. fat, 796 mg. calcium, 328 mg. sodium.

Lunch: Pear Quinoa Salad (leftover from Day 22), ½ Raspberry Smoothie.

Dinner: Filet Mignon, Roasted Brussels Sprouts with Cranberries and Walnuts, Sautéed Swiss Chard, Orange or Fruit of Choice.

Filet Mignon Recipe:

Per Person: Serving size is 4 ounces – cook enough to have 2 ounces left for Lunch Salad tomorrow.

Prepare Filet Mignon according to your preferred cooking method and doneness.

Optional: Cut garlic clove in half and rub filet with garlic or press finely chopped garlic into top of filet. Season filet with freshly ground black pepper.

Roasted Brussels Sprouts with Cranberries and Walnuts Recipe: Serves 2.
Preheat oven to 400° F.

8 ounces Brussels Sprouts
1 tsp. olive oil
¼ tsp. sea salt
1 Tbsp. balsamic vinegar
1 tsp. chopped fresh thyme
1 Tbsp. dried cranberries
1 Tbsp. chopped walnuts
2 Tbsp. Gorgonzola cheese, crumbled

Cut ends off Brussels sprouts and then cut in half. Carefully coat sprouts with olive oil and salt. It works best if you use your hands. Evenly distribute sprouts on parchment lined baking sheet and cook for 15 to 20 minutes at 400° F. or until tender. Stir half way through cooking time. Remove from oven when done.

Coat sprouts with balsamic vinegar. Stir in thyme, dried cranberries and walnuts. Top with cheese.

Nutritional analysis per serving: 141 calories, 6 g. protein, 5 g. fiber, 8 g. fat, 101 mg. calcium, 440 mg. sodium.

Sautéed Swiss Chard Recipe:

Per person:
In skillet over medium heat sauté 3 cups Swiss chard in 1 tsp. olive oil until tender. Add black pepper to taste. May also add fresh lemon juice if desired.

Nutritional analysis per serving: 60 calories, 2 g. protein, 2 g. fiber, 5 g. fat, 55 mg. calcium, 230 mg. sodium.

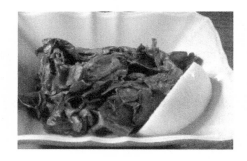

Day 25 Menu

Breakfast
Ricotta English Muffin with Strawberries
1 Egg cooked any way
Beverage of Choice

Lunch
Steak and Rice Bowl
2 squares 85% Dark Chocolate
½ cup Raspberries
Beverage of Choice

Dinner
Sweet Potato Carrot Soup
Massaged Kale Salad
1 serving Whole Grain Bread
Beverage of Choice

If restricting sodium to 1500 mg/day: May not add salt or soy sauce to food or in cooking beyond what is already in the recipes.
2300 mg/day: May not add additional salt to food or in cooking - may use 1 Tbsp. low sodium soy sauce on Steak and Rice Bowl.

If not restricting calories to 1600/day:
Lunch: May have 2 extra ounces of steak in salad and a serving whole grain bread.
Dinner: May have extra soup.

Recipes
Breakfast: Ricotta English Muffin with Strawberries, 1 Egg cooked any way.

English Muffin with Ricotta Cheese and Sliced Strawberries:

For each serving:
1 Whole grain English muffin
½ cup ricotta cheese
1 tsp. honey
4 medium strawberries, sliced

Split English muffin in half and toast if desired. Mix ricotta cheese with honey and spread evenly over 2 English muffin halves. Layer strawberries on top of cheese mixture.

Nutritional analysis per serving: 342 calories, 20 g. protein, 5 g. fiber, 11 g. fat, 520 mg. calcium, 396 mg. sodium.

Lunch: Steak & Rice Bowl, 2 squares 85% Dark Chocolate, ½ cup Raspberries.

Steak and Rice Bowl Recipe:

Per person:
2 ounces filet mignon, sliced (leftover from yesterday's dinner)
¼ cup uncooked brown rice
1 cup mushrooms, sliced – any type or mix of types and can use
  more than 1 cup, if desired
2 cups raw spinach
2 tsp. olive oil, divided
1 green onion, chopped
Low sodium soy sauce – no soy sauce if limiting sodium to 1500
  mg./day, may have 1 Tbsp. if limiting sodium to 2300 mg./day.

Cook brown rice according to package directions. Keep warm.

Sauté mushrooms in 1 tsp. olive oil until tender. Sauté spinach in 1 tsp. olive oil until just wilted.

Put warm brown rice in bowl. Top rice with mushrooms, spinach, green onion and steak. Add soy sauce.

Nutritional analysis per serving without soy sauce: 371 calories, 23 g. protein, 4 g. fiber, 15 g. fat, 82 mg. calcium, 87 mg. sodium.

With 1 Tbsp. soy sauce serving is approximately 620 mg. sodium.

Dinner: Sweet Potato Carrot Soup, Massaged Kale Salad, 1 serving Whole Grain Bread.

Sweet Potato Carrot Soup Recipe: Makes 5 servings – make enough for Dinner and Lunch the next day - you can freeze any additional leftovers for another time.

2 pounds carrots, sliced
2 sweet potatoes, cut into chunks
2 quarts low sodium vegetable broth
2 cups water
1/8 tsp. sea salt
1 cup white wine (optional – may substitute water)
1 Tbsp. turmeric
2 15-ounce cans (3 ½ cups) white beans (Navy, Cannellini) I like
    Eden No Salt Added canned beans with BPA free lining or try
    Whole Foods 365 Organic No salt added beans that are packed
    in cartons. If you have time cook your own from dried beans.
½ cup plus 2 Tbsp. grated Parmesan cheese

In a large pot, mix carrots, sweet potatoes, vegetable broth, water, salt, white wine, turmeric and white beans (if using canned beans do not drain beans – if not using canned add 1 cup of water in addition to water already in recipe). Bring mixture to a boil over medium high heat, then reduce heat to medium and simmer until carrots and sweet potatoes are tender, about 1 hour.

In batches transfer soup to blender and blend until smooth. CAUTION: Blending hot liquids will cause the lid of the blender to explode off. To avoid burns and a mess only fill the blender half full (blend in batches) and vent the lid. Many blenders have a lid with a center piece that comes out. Remove the center piece. Cover lid with kitchen towel to avoid sprays but still allow steam to escape. May use immersion blender instead.

Serve with 2 Tbsp. grated Parmesan cheese on top of each bowl of soup.

Nutritional analysis per serving: 384 calories, 24 g. protein, 14 g. fiber, 8 g. fat, 263 mg. calcium, 562 mg. sodium.

Massaged Kale Salad Recipe:

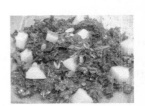

Per person:
4 cups fresh, raw kale – washed and dried
2 tsp. olive oil, divided
1/8 tsp. sea salt
1 Tbsp. lemon juice plus 2 tsp. lemon juice
1 tsp. honey
½ mango
1 tsp. pumpkin seeds

Remove the ribs and slice or tear the kale into bite size pieces (the kale will shrink as you massage it). Add the kale, 1 tsp. olive oil, salt and 1 Tbsp. lemon juice to a bowl. Massage kale with both hands. Massage 2 to 5 minutes, tasting it as you massage to get it to the texture and flavor you like. The longer you massage the more tender and less bitter the kale becomes.

In a separate bowl or jar mix honey, 2 tsp. lemon juice and 1 tsp. olive oil until smooth. Shake all ingredients in a jar or mix lemon juice and olive oil in a small bowl with a whisk until smooth, then whisk in olive oil until well blended. Add dressing to kale.

Top kale with mango slices and pumpkin seeds.

If not restricting calories to 1600/day may use more olive oil, mango and pumpkin seeds.

Nutritional Analysis for 1 serving: 323 calories, 13 grams protein, 8 grams fiber, 13 grams fat, 417 mg. calcium, 396 mg sodium.

Day 26 Menu

Breakfast
Smoked Salmon and Arugula Omelet
Whole Grain Toast
Citrus with Kiwi
Beverage of Choice

Snack anytime during the Day
½ Peach Smoothie

Lunch
Sweet Potato Carrot Soup
½ Peach Smoothie
Beverage of Choice

Dinner
Portobello Mushroom Tacos
Balsamic Strawberries with Greek Yogurt
Beverage of Choice

If restricting sodium to 1500 mg/day: May not add salt to food or in cooking beyond what is already in the recipes - will need to use corn tortillas or low sodium flour tortillas for tacos.
2300 mg/day: May not add additional salt to food or in cooking - may use regular flour tortillas for tacos.

If not restricting calories to 1600/day:
Breakfast: May have second slice of toast or biscuits.
Lunch: May have extra soup and a serving of whole grain bread.
Dinner: May have extra tacos, avocado or guacamole and extra Balsamic Strawberries.

Recipes
Breakfast: Smoked Salmon and Arugula Omelet, Whole Grain Toast, Citrus with Kiwi.

Smoked Salmon and Arugula Omelet Recipe:

Per Person:
1 tsp. olive oil, divided
2 cups arugula – may substitute spinach if you prefer a milder green
2 large eggs (may substitute 4 egg whites or 1 egg plus 2 egg
   whites)
Dash of black pepper
1 green onion, chopped
1 ounce smoked salmon, chopped
1 Tbsp. cream cheese
Sliced tomato

Heat ½ tsp. olive oil in skillet over medium heat. Sauté arugula until just wilted. Keep warm.

Beat eggs in bowl with black pepper and green onion. The smoked salmon gives the dish plenty of saltiness so there is no need for additional salt.

Heat ½ tsp. olive oil in skillet over low heat. Add eggs and prepare omelet over low heat, adding smoked salmon, cream cheese and arugula to one half of the omelet once eggs are almost done. Fold omelet in half by folding half without fillings over half with salmon mixture. Cook until eggs are just done (I like to put a lid on the pan to finish cooking the eggs). (If you prefer you can do this recipe as scrambled eggs, mixing in salmon, cream cheese and arugula when eggs are almost done). Serve immediately with sliced tomato.

Nutritional analysis per serving: 261 calories, 20 g. protein, 1 g. fiber, 18 g. fat, 151 mg. calcium, 448 mg. sodium.

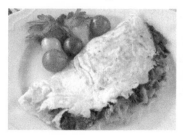

Citrus with Kiwi Recipe:

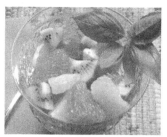

Per person:
½ orange, sectioned
½ grapefruit, sectioned
½ kiwi, sliced
Fresh mint leaves (optional)

Mix fruit together. Garnish with fresh mint or basil leaves if desired.

Nutritional analysis per serving: 95 calories, 2 g. protein, 4 g. fiber, 0 g. fat, 54 mg. calcium, 1 mg. sodium.

Lunch: Sweet Potato Carrot Soup (leftover from yesterday), ½ Peach Smoothie.

Peach Smoothie Recipe: Drink ½ with Lunch and ½ as a snack. Per person blend all of the following ingredients in a high-speed blender until smooth:
¾ cup of unsweetened Almond Milk (Calcium calculation based on using almond milk containing 300 mg calcium per 8 ounces or 30% of the calcium RDA. If using a product higher than 300 mg. then use only amount of Almond Milk required for 300 mg. calcium and use water for the rest of the liquid).
¼ cup plain nonfat Greek Yogurt (containing 300 mg calcium per 1 cup serving. Nutrition label will say 30% of the RDA for calcium)
1 cup raw kale
1/2 cup frozen or fresh peach slices (may substitute another fruit for peach)
1 medium banana
1 Tbsp. flaxseed (optional, just adds 37 calories and has lots of health benefits)

Add additional water or ice cubes if a different consistency is desired. If you have parsley or other greens that you need to use before they go bad then add them to your smoothie – don't let them go to waste. If not restricting calories to 1600 per day you may add additional fruits and vegetables as desired.
Nutritional analysis for 1 Smoothie not including flaxseed: 249 calories, 12 g. protein, 7 g. fiber, 4 g. fat, 414 mg. calcium, 185 mg. sodium.

Dinner: Portobello Mushroom Tacos, Balsamic Strawberries with Greek Yogurt.

Portobello Mushroom Tacos Recipe: Makes 4 Tacos, 2 per serving – prepare enough ingredients to have for Dinner today and Lunch tomorrow.

Preheat oven to 400° F.

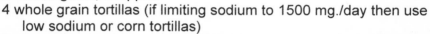

20 cherry tomatoes
2 ½ tsp. olive oil, divided
2 Portobello Mushrooms
¼ cup chopped red onion
¼ tsp. black pepper, or to taste
2 cloves garlic, chopped
4 whole grain tortillas (if limiting sodium to 1500 mg./day then use
     low sodium or corn tortillas)
Salsa or hot sauce of choice, I like a verde or green salsa with these
Avocado or Guacamole (optional and if not limiting calories to
     1600/day)

In bowl mix tomatoes with ½ tsp. olive oil.   Spread tomatoes evenly on a baking sheet lined with parchment paper and roast at 400° F. for 15 minutes or until tomatoes split and pop.   Remove from oven and set aside.   Reduce heat to 350°.

Wrap tortillas in foil and warm in 350 °F. oven. (or use whatever method you prefer for warming tortillas).

Remove stems from Portobello mushrooms.   Wipe Portobello mushrooms clean and quickly rinse under cold water.   Dry with a paper towel.   Cut Portobello mushrooms into thin length wise pieces or if you prefer bite size pieces.   Heat olive oil in skillet over medium heat.   Sauté mushrooms and onion in olive oil until tender.   Add black pepper, garlic and tomatoes and cook for 1 minute.   Serve in warm tortillas with salsa.   If you can afford the extra calories add some avocado chunks or guacamole to the tacos.

Nutrient analysis for 2 tacos without the avocado: 341 calories, 13 g. fat, 10 g. protein, 6 g. fiber, 32 mg. calcium, 898 mg. sodium.

1/4th of an avocado adds 80 calories, 1 g. protein, 3 g. fiber, 7 g. fat, 6 mg. calcium and 4 mg. sodium.

Balsamic Strawberries with Greek Yogurt Recipe:

Per person:
1 cup strawberries, sliced
1 Tbsp. balsamic vinegar
¾ cup plain, nonfat Greek Yogurt
1 tsp. honey

In bowl mix strawberries with balsamic vinegar.   In a separate bowl mix Greek yogurt with honey.   In a parfait, or similar type glass, layer strawberries with Greek yogurt mixture.

Nutritional analysis per serving: 182 calories, 18 g. protein, 3 g. fiber, 0 g. fat, 253 mg. calcium, 76 mg. sodium.

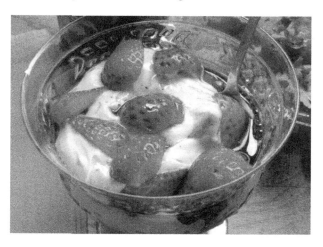

Day 27 Menu

Breakfast
Blueberry Whole Wheat Pancakes
1/2 Pineapple Smoothie
Beverage of Choice

Lunch
Portobello Mushroom Tacos
1 Orange or Fruit of choice
1/2 Pineapple Smoothie
Beverage of Choice

Dinner
Quail (or Chicken Breast) with Fig Glaze
Sautéed Mushrooms
Apple Arugula Salad with Maple Lemon Dressing
Beverage of Choice

If restricting sodium to 1500 mg/day: Use corn tortillas or low sodium flour tortillas at Lunch and may have 1/16th tsp. salt added to food or in cooking beyond what is already in the recipes.
2300 mg/day: May use regular tortillas for tacos and may add scant ¼ tsp. salt to food or in cooking.

If not restricting calories to 1600/day:
Breakfast: May have extra pancakes and 1 egg.
Lunch: May have extra tacos and avocado.
Dinner: May have a second quail, a serving whole grain bread and additional Tbsp. goat cheese on salad.

Recipes:
<u>**Breakfast:**</u>   Blueberry Whole Wheat Pancakes, ½ Pineapple Smoothie.

Blueberry Whole Wheat Pancakes Recipe: Makes Eight 4-½ inch pancakes.   Serving size, if limiting calories to 1600/day, is 2 pancakes.

1 egg
1 cup buttermilk
2 Tbsp. canola oil – preferably organic or non-GMO
1 cup whole wheat flour
1 Tbsp. sugar
1 tsp. baking powder
½ tsp. baking soda
¼ tsp. salt
1 tsp. vanilla
½ tsp. cinnamon
3 cups blueberries, fresh or frozen - divided
2 cups applesauce

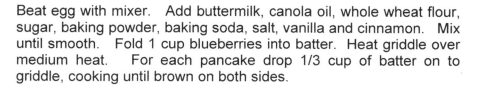

Beat egg with mixer.   Add buttermilk, canola oil, whole wheat flour, sugar, baking powder, baking soda, salt, vanilla and cinnamon.   Mix until smooth.   Fold 1 cup blueberries into batter. Heat griddle over medium heat.   For each pancake drop 1/3 cup of batter on to griddle, cooking until brown on both sides.

Top each pancake with ¼ cup applesauce and ¼ cup blueberries. If not limiting calories to 1600/day and you feel the need for maple syrup, a good way to cut down on amount of syrup used is to mix a little syrup with the applesauce and top with blueberries.

Nutritional analysis for 2 pancakes (without maple syrup):   333 calories, 8 g. protein, 8 g. fiber, 10 g. fat, 174 mg. calcium, 511 mg. sodium.

Pineapple Smoothie Recipe: Drink ½ with Breakfast and ½ with Lunch.

Per person blend all of the following ingredients in a high-speed blender until smooth:

¾ cup of unsweetened Almond Milk (Calcium calculation based on using almond milk containing 300 mg calcium per 8 ounces or 30% of the calcium RDA. If using a product higher than 300 mg. then use only amount of Almond Milk required for 300 mg. calcium and use water for the rest of the liquid).
1 cup plain nonfat Greek Yogurt (containing 300 mg calcium per 1 cup serving. Nutrition label will say 30% of the RDA for calcium)
1 1/2 cup raw kale
1 cup frozen, canned or fresh pineapple (may substitute another fruit for pineapple)
1 medium banana
1 Tbsp. flaxseed (optional, just adds 37 calories and has lots of health benefits)

Add additional water or ice cubes if a different consistency is desired. If you have parsley or other greens that you need to use before they go bad then add them to your smoothie – don't let them go to waste. If not restricting calories to 1600 per day you may add additional fruits and vegetables as desired.

Nutritional analysis per serving not including flaxseed: 389 calories, 30 g. protein, 6 g. fiber, 4 g. fat, 703 mg. calcium, 271 mg. sodium.

Lunch: Portobello Mushroom Tacos (leftover from yesterday's dinner), 1 Orange or fruit of choice, 1/2 Pineapple Smoothie.

Dinner: Quail (or Chicken Breast) with Fig Glaze, Sautéed Mushrooms, Apple Arugula Salad with Maple Lemon Dressing.

Quail with Fig Glaze Recipe:
If baking quail, instead of grilling, preheat oven to 350° F.

Per Person:
1 Tbsp. Fig Preserves
1/2 tsp. brandy

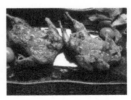

Orange juice
1 Quail (may substitute 4 ounce chicken breast)
Olive oil - about ½ tsp. per quail
Black Pepper, as desired
1/8 tsp. ground cinnamon
1/8 tsp. ground cloves
1/8 tsp. ground ginger

For glaze, in small bowl mix fig preserves with brandy. Add enough orange juice, 1 to 3 tsp., to get glaze to desired consistency. The amount you need depends on the thickness of your jam.

Lightly rub quail on both sides and under skin with olive oil, black pepper, cinnamon, cloves and ginger.   Brush lightly with glaze. Grill or bake quail (or chicken) until done. If grilling quail, cooking time should be 3 to 5 minutes depending on how hot your grill is. If baking quail, bake 10 to 15 minutes or until done, in a 350° F. oven. Top with remaining glaze and serve. May warm glaze or serve at room temperature.

Nutritional analysis per person: 265 calories, 21 g. protein, 12 g. fat, 18 mg. calcium, 44 mg. sodium.

Sautéed Mushrooms Recipe:

Per person:
1 cup mushrooms, cleaned, stems trimmed, sliced
1 tsp. olive oil
1 Tbsp. White wine
1 tsp. fresh or ½ tsp. dried Thyme
1/8 tsp. black pepper, or to taste

In skillet, heat olive oil over medium high heat. Add mushrooms and cook, stirring frequently, until mushrooms release liquid.   Then increase heat to high and cook, stirring frequently, until liquid from mushrooms evaporates. Reduce heat to medium and add white wine and continue to cook until mushrooms are tender and wine has evaporated. Sprinkle with thyme and pepper then serve.

Nutritional analysis per serving: 54 calories, 2 g. protein, 1 g. fiber, 5 mg. fat, 2 mg. calcium, 4 mg. sodium.

Apple Arugula Salad Recipe:

For each person mix:
2 cups arugula (may substitute other greens)
½ apple (if making salad for 1 go ahead and eat the whole apple if
    you like)
4 endive leaves (may substitute escarole or romaine lettuce)
2 Tbsp. Maple Lemon Dressing – recipe below

Top with:
1 Tbsp. chopped toasted walnuts
1 Tbsp. Pomegranate arils (optional)
1 Tbsp. goat cheese

Maple Lemon Dressing:
Mix the following ingredients together in a jar and shake until well
blended:
2 Tbsp. maple syrup
¼ cup fresh lemon juice
1 Tbsp. Dijon mustard
¼ cup olive oil

Nutritional Analysis for 1 serving salad with 2 Tbsp. dressing: 252
calories, 5 g. protein, 4 g. fiber, 17 g. fat, 129 mg. calcium, 61 mg.
sodium.

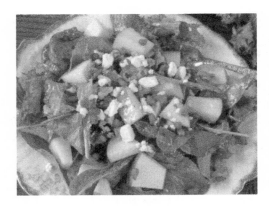

Day 28 Menu

Breakfast
Fried Eggs on Wilted Kale
Broiled Tomato Halves
Whole Grain Toast with 1 Tbsp. Jam
Beverage of Choice

Snack Anytime during the Day
3 cups Popcorn
½ Blueberry Smoothie

Lunch
Shrimp Cocktail
½ Blueberry Smoothie
Beverage of Choice

Dinner
Zin Spaghetti with Roasted Vegetables
Garlic Toast
Beverage of Choice

If restricting sodium to 1500 mg/day: Do not add salt to food or in cooking beyond what is already in the recipes and leave the salt out of the Zin Spaghetti.
2300 mg/day: may add a scant ¼ tsp. salt to food or in cooking

If not restricting calories to 1600/day:
Breakfast: May have second slice of toast or whole grain biscuits.
Snack: May have 6 cups popcorn.
Dinner: May have additional Zin spaghetti.

Recipes:

Breakfast: Fried Eggs on Wilted Kale, Broiled Tomato Halves, Whole Grain Toast with 1 Tbsp. Jam.

Fried Eggs on Wilted Kale Recipe:

Per person:
2 eggs
2 tsp. olive oil - divided
2 cups kale (may use more kale if desired)
Black pepper

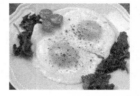

In skillet heat 1 tsp. olive oil over medium heat. Cook kale just until wilted. Keep warm.

Fry eggs in remaining 1 tsp. olive oil.

Serve eggs on top of kale. Add black pepper as desired.

Nutritional analysis per serving: 288 calories, 18 g. protein, 3 g. fiber, 19 g. fat, 257 mg. calcium, 193 mg. sodium.

Broiled Tomato halves Recipe:

Turn oven to broil
Per person:
1 tomato
Cinnamon, ground
Allspice. ground
Red wine vinegar

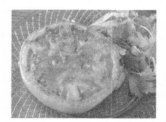

Cut tomato in half. Place cut side up on baking pan. Brush top of tomato halves with red wine vinegar and sprinkle with cinnamon and allspice. Broil until warm and desired texture and doneness, about 5 minutes.

Nutritional analysis per serving: 22 calories, 1 g. protein, 1 g. fiber, .25 g fat, 12 mg calcium, 6 mg sodium.

Lunch: Shrimp Cocktail, ½ Blueberry Smoothie.

Shrimp Cocktail Recipe: Makes 2 servings.

6 ounces cooked shrimp - Go to www.seafoodwatch.org for
 sustainable fish purchasing guidelines.   You can also look for
 fish with the Marine Stewardship Council Blue eco-label in your
 grocery store.
12 cherry tomatoes, cut in half
2 jalapeno peppers, finely chopped (use less if you like less heat)
2 Tbsp. chopped cilantro
½ cup pineapple chunks or tidbits, drained if from can
Avocado, if not limiting calories to 1600 per day

In bowl mix shrimp, tomatoes, jalapeno, cilantro and pineapple. If
not limiting calories to 1600 per day add avocado chunks.   Serve
chilled.

Nutrient analysis per serving without avocado added: 191 calories,
25 g. protein, 2 g. fiber, 2 g. fat, 85 mg. calcium, 511 mg. sodium.

1/4th of an avocado adds 80 calories, 1 g. protein, 3 g. fiber, 7 g. fat,
6 mg. calcium and 4 mg. sodium.

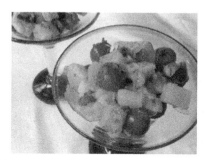

Blueberry Smoothie Recipe: Drink ½ with Lunch and ½ as a
snack anytime during the day.

Per person blend all of the following ingredients in a high-speed
blender until smooth:

1 ½ cup of unsweetened Almond Milk (Calcium calculation based on

using almond milk containing 300 mg calcium per 8 ounces or 30% of the calcium RDA. If using a product higher than 300 mg. then use only amount of Almond Milk required for 300 mg. calcium and use water for the rest of the liquid).
2 cups raw spinach
1 cup frozen or fresh blueberries (may substitute another fruit for blueberries)
1 medium banana
1 Tbsp. flaxseed (optional, just adds 37 calories and has lots of health benefits)

Add additional water or ice cubes if a different consistency is desired. If you have parsley or other greens that you need to use before they go bad then add them to your smoothie – don't let them go to waste. If not limiting calories to 1600 per day may add additional fruits and vegetables as desired.

Nutritional analysis per Smoothie: 258 calories, 5 g. protein, 10 g. fiber, 6 g. fat, 528 mg. calcium, 320 mg. sodium.

Snack anytime: 3 cups Popcorn, ½ Blueberry Smoothie.

Dinner: Zin Spaghetti with Roasted Vegetables, Garlic Toast.

Zin Spaghetti with Roasted Vegetables Recipe:

Serves 4
Preheat oven to 400° F.

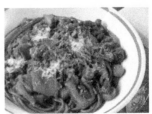

1 Eggplant, cut into bite size cubes
2 Tbsp. olive oil, divided
1 tsp. smoked paprika
½ tsp. garlic powder
3 medium carrots, sliced into bite size pieces
1 red bell pepper, sliced into bite size pieces
8 ounces mushrooms, left whole
1 cup cherry tomatoes
1/8 tsp. cayenne pepper
1 15 ounce can no salt added black beans – drained (or 1 ¾ cup cooked black beans, drained)

½ tsp. sea salt, divided (leave salt out if limiting sodium to 1500
  mg./day)
3 Tbsp. low salt/sodium tomato paste, divided
¼ tsp. black pepper
1 tsp. crushed red pepper, divided
¼ cup fresh oregano, or 1 Tbsp. dried oregano
8 ounces whole grain spaghetti
3 cloves garlic, chopped
1 shallot, chopped
2 cups Red Zinfandel wine (see directions below if you don't want to
  use the wine)
¼ cup flat leaf parsley, chopped
½ cup freshly grated Parmesan cheese

Mix eggplant with 1 tsp. olive oil, smoked paprika and garlic powder.
Evenly distribute eggplant on a parchment lined baking sheet. Mix
carrots and red bell pepper with 2 tsp. olive oil and evenly distribute
on a parchment lined baking sheet. Mix mushrooms and 1 tsp. olive
oil and evenly distribute on a parchment lined baking sheet. Mix
tomatoes with 1 tsp. olive oil and cayenne pepper. Evenly distribute
tomatoes on a parchment lined baking pan. Roast vegetables at
400° F.

Cherry tomatoes should be done in 15 to 20 minutes (just after they
start to split or pop open). Eggplant should be done in about 25
minutes. Mushrooms should be done in about 30 minutes. Carrots
and bell pepper should be done in about 40 minutes.

Bring pot of water to a boil. Add pasta and cook until almost done.
Drain well.

Mix roasted vegetables together in a large saucepan. Carefully mix
in black beans. Mix in ¼ tsp. salt, 2 Tbsp. tomato paste, ¼ tsp.
black pepper, ½ tsp. crushed red pepper and oregano. Keep warm
over low heat.

In a large skillet, heat 1 tsp. olive oil over medium heat. Add garlic,
½ tsp. red pepper, and shallot. Sauté for 30 seconds. Add wine, ¼
tsp. salt and 1 Tbsp. tomato paste. Add drained spaghetti. Simmer
over medium heat, stirring frequently, for 3 to 4 minutes or until most
of wine is absorbed and pasta is done.

(If you don't want to use red wine then cook the spaghetti according to package directions until done, drain well and mix in 1 tsp. olive oil, garlic, ½ tsp. red pepper, shallot, ¼ tsp. salt and 1 Tbsp. tomato paste. Mix to coat spaghetti).
Divide pasta into serving bowls and top with vegetable bean mixture. Then top with parsley and 2 Tbsp. Parmesan cheese per serving. Serve with 1 slice of Garlic toast limiting butter on toast to 1 tsp. if limiting calories to 1600/day.

Nutritional Analysis per serving: 507 calories, 13 g. fat, 24 g. protein, 13 g. fiber, 269 mg calcium, 549 mg. sodium. If leave salt out of recipe sodium will be 259 mg.

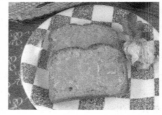

Garlic Toast Recipe:

Per serving:
1 slice 100% whole grain bread
1 tsp. unsalted butter, softened
Fresh garlic, finely chopped or mashed (may substitute garlic
    powder)

Spread butter evenly over bread. Sprinkle garlic on top of bread. Broil or toast until browned. Serve immediately.

A tasty option is to roast the garlic and spread the roasted garlic over the bread. The roasted garlic has a creamy texture and can be spread on the bread just like butter – so good you don't even need the butter. To roast garlic, remove papery skin from garlic head but do not separate the garlic cloves from the head. Cut off tip ends of cloves so it will be easier to squeeze garlic out. Place garlic in small oven safe bowl or pan. Pour 1 tsp. olive oil over garlic head coating all the cloves and cover with foil. Cook at 400° F. until garlic is soft when pressed, about 30 to 40 minutes. Remove from oven and allow to cool. Once cool enough to work with squeeze garlic out of skins and spread on bread.

Nutritional analysis for 1 slice whole grain garlic bread with unsalted butter (may vary according to bread you use): 111 calories, 4 g. protein, 2 g. fiber, 5 g. fat, 34 mg. calcium, 124 mg. sodium.

Appendix A
Protein Needs for Strength Training

Your protein requirement will be higher if you are engaged in a strength-training program to build muscle and strengthen your bones. You will also burn more calories when engaged in a regular exercise program.

Strength training is any exercise that uses some form of resistance to strengthen and build muscle. Strength training includes using hand-held weights, weight machines, resistance bands, resistance balls and your own body to develop muscle. Research shows that strength training can dramatically reduce fracture risk in postmenopausal women. Women who regularly strength train also have been shown to gain bone strength in their hip and spine as well as improving their balance. Women with osteoporosis or osteopenia should consult with their doctor prior to starting a strength-training program and be sure to work with a trainer or physical therapist specifically trained in programs for people with osteoporosis. If you undertake a strength-training program then you need to be sure you are eating enough protein to maximize muscle synthesis while still keeping a good acid alkaline balance in your diet.

In general, recreational adult exercisers need 0.5 to 0.7 grams of protein per pound of body weight. Adults working to build muscle mass with strength training need 0.7 to 0.8 grams of protein per pound of body weight. If you are overweight calculate your protein needs using your ideal body weight instead of your actual weight. For example, to calculate the strength training protein requirement of a person weighing 125 pounds, that is not overweight; multiply 125 by .8 to get 100 grams protein per day. Or, for overweight individual with an ideal body weight of 115 pounds, multiply 115 by .8 to get 92 grams protein per day.

The eating plan evenly distributes protein at all 3 meals (25 to 30 grams protein per meal) of the day and averages around 80 grams of protein per day. To determine your additional protein needs for strength training subtract 80 grams from your required protein amount. For example, if your strength training protein need is for 100 grams protein then subtract 80 from 100 to get a need for 20 additional grams of protein per day. Consume some of the additional protein as a post workout snack within 45 minutes of finishing your workout. If you eat breakfast, lunch or dinner within 45 minutes of working out then add your extra protein as in between meal snacks during the day. It is important to spread your protein intake out during the day and not eat the bulk of your protein at one or two meals or snacks. Your muscles need a steady supply of protein all day and in general most people can't absorb more than 25 to 30 grams of protein at one time. You also must consume adequate calories from carbohydrates and healthy fats so that protein is available for optimal utilization by the body.

A good way to get the extra protein and still maintain a good alkaline acid balance in your diet is to drink a high protein smoothie made with Greek yogurt, fruits and vegetables, or eat cottage or ricotta cheese with fruit, or nuts with dried fruit.

The following table outlines some protein options while following the Eating Plan:

Protein Option	Calories	Protein	Calcium	To balance out Acid:
Smoothie: 1 cup Greek Yogurt, 1 cup kale, 1 Banana, ½ cup fruit	Approx. 300	28 grams	Approx. 400 mg	Already balanced -Fruits and kale in smoothie balance out acid from yogurt
½ cup skim milk cottage cheese	50	8 grams	62 mg	Eat ½ serving of fruit or vegetable
½ cup part skim ricotta cheese	160	10 grams	400 mg	Eat ½ serving of fruit or vegetable
½ cup fat free plain Greek yogurt	65	12 grams	150 mg	Eat ½ serving of fruit or vegetable
1 large boiled egg	72	6 grams	28 mg	Eat 1 serving of fruit or vegetable
2 Tbsp. unsalted unsweetened almond butter	197	7 grams	111 mg	
2 Tbsp. unsalted peanut butter	188	8 grams	14 mg	Eat 1 serving of fruit or vegetable
½ cup Edamame, unsalted	65	6 grams	35 mg	
1 cup skim milk	83	8 grams	299 mg	Eat 1 serving fruit or vegetable
1 cup soy milk	131	8 grams	61 mg	Eat 1 serving fruit or vegetable
1 Babybel Mozzarella cheese	50	6 grams	200 mg	Eat 1 serving fruit or vegetable
¼ cup goat cheese	126	8 grams	155 mg	Eat 1 serving fruit or vegetable
1 oz mozzarella cheese	106	7 grams	212 mg	Eat 2 servings fruit or vegetable
1 oz provolone cheese	100	7 grams	214 mg	Eat 2 servings fruit or vegetable
1 oz muenster cheese	104	7 grams	203 mg	Eat 2 servings fruit or vegetable
1 oz cheddar cheese	114	7 grams	204 mg	Eat 2 servings fruit or vegetable
1 ounce chicken breast	47	7 grams	3 mg	Eat 1 serving fruit or vegetable
1 ounce lean roast beef	56	8 grams	2 mg	Eat 1 serving fruit or vegetable
1 ounce pork tenderloin	42	7 grams	2 mg	Eat 1 serving fruit or vegetable
2 ounces (about ¼ cup) tuna packed in water, no salt added	66	15 grams	6 mg	Eat 1 serving fruit or vegetable
¼ cup hummus	102	5 grams	23 mg	Eat ½ serving fruit or vegetable
1 ounce or 14 walnut halves, un salted	185	4 grams	28 mg	Eat 1 serving fruit or vegetable
¼ cup dry roasted no salt added pistachios	174	6 grams	33 mg	Eat 1 serving fruit or vegetable
¼ cup unsalted whole almond	208	8 grams	96 mg	

1 serving of a fruit or vegetable is ½ cup, or for raw greens, 1 cup.

INDEX

Made in the USA
Las Vegas, NV
03 June 2023